W9-CBS-268

PRACTICAL
GUIDE
SERIES

CDT 2014

Dental Procedure Codes

ADA American Dental Association®

America's leading advocate for oral health

Table of Contents

© 2013 American Dental Association

Preface

Introduction

This reference manual, published by the ADA, contains the *Code on Dental Procedures and Nomenclature* (CDT Code) version that is effective for services provided on or after January 1, 2014 through December 31, 2014.

In August 2000 the CDT Code was designated by the federal government as the national terminology for reporting dental services on claims submitted to third-party payers, in accordance with authority granted by the Health Insurance Portability and Accountability Act of 1996 (HIPAA).

The ADA's Council on Dental Benefit Programs is responsible for maintaining the CDT Code in accordance with ADA Bylaws and policy, and applicable federal regulations. CDT Manual content is developed by the Council, while responsibility for CDT Manual printing, pricing and distribution of falls to the ADA's Department of Product Development and Sales.

- Should you have any recommendations for **additions, revisions or deletions** to the CDT Code, direct access to the process is available via the portal established on the ADA web page *www.ada.org/3827.aspx*.

- **Technical questions** on the CDT Code or ADA Dental Claim Form should be directed to the ADA's Member Service Center (members: toll free number on your membership card; non-members: 312-440-2500).

- For general information about, or to pursue CDT Code **licensing,** please go to the ADA web page *www.ada.org/3854.aspx*. In addition to information about licensing this site contains the questionnaire that must be completed as the first step of the licensing process.

- For any questions regarding **pricing or purchasing** additional copies of the CDT Manual visit *www.adacatalog.org* or call 800-947-4746.

Preface

Categories of Service

The CDT Code is organized into twelve categories of service, each with its own series of five-digit alphanumeric codes:

Category of Service	Code Series
I. Diagnostic	D0100 – D0999
II. Preventive	D1000 – D1999
III. Restorative	D2000 – D2999
IV. Endodontics	D3000 – D3999
V. Periodontics	D4000 – D4999
VI. Prosthodontics, removable	D5000 – D5899
VII. Maxillofacial Prosthetics	D5900 – D5999
VIII. Implant Services	D6000 – D6199
IX. Prosthodontics, fixed	D6200 – D6999
X. Oral & Maxillofacial Surgery	D7000 – D7999
XI. Orthodontics	D8000 – D8999
XII. Adjunctive General Services	D9000 – D9999

These categories exist solely as a means to organize the CDT Code. As a result, some categories of service are divided into subcategories of related procedures. Many categories and subcategories have descriptors applicable to all procedure codes therein.

Dental procedure codes within a Category of Service, or a subcategory, are not always in numeric order. The reason is that existing numeric sequences often do not have unassigned codes available for CDT Code additions.

 © 2013 American Dental Association

Components of a Dental Procedure Code Entry

Every procedure in the CDT Code must have the first two of the following three components:

1. **Procedure Code** – A five character alphanumeric code beginning with the letter "D" that identifies a specific dental procedure. A Procedure Code cannot be changed or abbreviated.

2. **Nomenclature** – The written title of a Procedure Code. Nomenclature may be abbreviated when printed on claim forms or other documents that are subject to space limitation. Any such abbreviation does not constitute a change to the Nomenclature.

3. **Descriptor** – A written narrative that further defines the nature and intended use of a single Procedure Code, or group of such codes. A Descriptor, when present, follows the applicable Procedure Code and its Nomenclature. Descriptors that apply to a series of Procedure Codes precede that series of codes.

Preface

Using the CDT Code

The following points should prove helpful when using the CDT Code for recording services provided on the patient record, and when reporting procedures on a paper or electronic claim submission.

1. The presence of a CDT Code does not mean that the procedure is:
   a. endorsed by any entity or is considered a standard of care
   b. covered or reimbursed by a dental benefits plan

2. General practitioners, specialists, and other individuals may report any of the listed CDT Codes as long as they are acting within the scope of their state law.

3. CDT Codes that require inclusion of a narrative description on the claim have the words "by report" in their nomenclature.

4. "Unspecified... procedure, by report" codes are used when, in the opinion of the dentist, there is no other CDT Code entry that accurately describes the services provided the patient.

Required Statement

If there is more than one code in this edition that consists of a procedure and a dentist submits a claim under one of these codes, the payor may process the claim under any of these codes that is consistent with the payor's reimbursement policy.

 © 2013 American Dental Association

1 Code on Dental Procedures and Nomenclature

ADA American Dental Association®

America's leading advocate for oral health

Code on Dental Procedures and Nomenclature

The current version of the *Code on Dental Procedures and Nomenclature* (CDT Code) that follows is effective for the calendar year January 1, 2014 through December 31, 2014. There are a number of changes from the prior version, which are identified by the following symbols:

- New procedure code
- ▲ Revision to a nomenclature or descriptor

Dental procedure codes that are no longer valid are not present. Chapter 2 contains the summary of all additions, revisions and deletions effective January 1, 2014.

As noted in the "Preface" the CDT Code is divided into twelve Categories of Service, and each category begins at the top of a right-hand page in this section of the manual.

Please note that when a code's nomenclature includes a "by report" notation, a narrative explaining the treatment provided must be included with the claim submission.

Classification of Materials

Names of dental materials are included in numerous procedure nomenclatures within several Categories of Service (e.g., Restorative; Prosthodontics, fixed). The following list of dental materials is included in the CDT Code **solely to aid selection** of a procedure code applicable to the service provided.

Classification of Metals (Source: ADA Council on Scientific Affairs – online at: *www.ada.org/2190.aspx*)

The noble metal classification system has been adopted as a more precise method of reporting various alloys used in dentistry. The alloys are defined on the basis of the percentage of metal content.

CLASSIFICATION	REQUIREMENT
High Noble Alloys	Noble Metal Content ≥ 60% (gold+ platinum group*) and gold ≥ 40%
Titanium and Titanium Alloys	Titanium ≥ 85%
Noble Alloys	Noble Metal Content ≥ 25% (gold + platinum group*)
Predominantly Base Alloys	Noble Metal Content < 25% (gold + platinum group*)

* metals of the platinum group are platinum, palladium, rhodium, iridium, osmium and ruthenium

Porcelain/ceramic
Refers to pressed, fired, polished or milled materials containing predominantly inorganic refractory compounds including porcelains, glasses, ceramics, and glass–ceramics.

Resin
Refers to any resin-based composite, including fiber or ceramic reinforced polymer compounds.

● new procedure code   ▲ revision to a nomenclature or descriptor

D0100–D0999   I. Diagnostic

Clinical Oral Evaluations

The codes in this section recognize the cognitive skills necessary for patient evaluation. The collection and recording of some data and components of the dental examination may be delegated; however, the evaluation, which includes diagnosis and treatment planning, is the responsibility of the dentist. As with all ADA procedure codes, there is no distinction made between the evaluations provided by general practitioners and specialists. Report additional diagnostic and/or definitive procedures separately.

D0120   periodic oral evaluation – established patient
An evaluation performed on a patient of record to determine any changes in the patient's dental and medical health status since a previous comprehensive or periodic evaluation. This includes an oral cancer evaluation and periodontal screening where indicated, and may require interpretation of information acquired through additional diagnostic procedures. Report additional diagnostic procedures separately.

D0140   limited oral evaluation – problem focused
An evaluation limited to a specific oral health problem or complaint. This may require interpretation of information acquired through additional diagnostic procedures. Report additional diagnostic procedures separately. Definitive procedures may be required on the same date as the evaluation.

Typically, patients receiving this type of evaluation present with a specific problem and/or dental emergencies, trauma, acute infections, etc.

D0145   oral evaluation for a patient under three years of age and counseling with primary caregiver
Diagnostic services performed for a child under the age of three, preferably within the first six months of the eruption of the first primary tooth, including recording the oral and physical health history, evaluation of caries susceptibility, development of an appropriate preventive oral health regimen and communication with and counseling of the child's parent, legal guardian and/or primary caregiver.

D0150 **comprehensive oral evaluation – new or established patient**
Used by a general dentist and/or a specialist when evaluating a patient comprehensively. This applies to new patients; established patients who have had a significant change in health conditions or other unusual circumstances, by report, or established patients who have been absent from active treatment for three or more years. It is a thorough evaluation and recording of the extraoral and intraoral hard and soft tissues. It may require interpretation of information acquired through additional diagnostic procedures. Additional diagnostic procedures should be reported separately.

This includes an evaluation for oral cancer where indicated, the evaluation and recording of the patient's dental and medical history and a general health assessment. It may include the evaluation and recording of dental caries, missing or unerupted teeth, restorations, existing prostheses, occlusal relationships, periodontal conditions (including periodontal screening and/or charting), hard and soft tissue anomalies, etc.

D0160 **detailed and extensive oral evaluation – problem focused, by report**
A detailed and extensive problem focused evaluation entails extensive diagnostic and cognitive modalities based on the findings of a comprehensive oral evaluation. Integration of more extensive diagnostic modalities to develop a treatment plan for a specific problem is required. The condition requiring this type of evaluation should be described and documented.

Examples of conditions requiring this type of evaluation may include dentofacial anomalies, complicated perio-prosthetic conditions, complex temporomandibular dysfunction, facial pain of unknown origin, conditions requiring multi-disciplinary consultation, etc.

D0170 **re-evaluation – limited, problem focused (established patient; not post-operative visit)**
Assessing the status of a previously existing condition. For example:

- a traumatic injury where no treatment was rendered but patient needs follow-up monitoring;

- evaluation for undiagnosed continuing pain;

- soft tissue lesion requiring follow-up evaluation.

D0180 **comprehensive periodontal evaluation – new or established patient**

This procedure is indicated for patients showing signs or symptoms of periodontal disease and for patients with risk factors such as smoking or diabetes. It includes evaluation of periodontal conditions, probing and charting, evaluation and recording of the patient's dental and medical history and general health assessment. It may include the evaluation and recording of dental caries, missing or unerupted teeth, restorations, occlusal relationships and oral cancer evaluation.

Pre-diagnostic Services

D0190 **screening of a patient**

A screening, including state or federally mandated screenings, to determine an individual's need to be seen by a dentist for diagnosis.

D0191 **assessment of a patient**

A limited clinical inspection that is performed to identify possible signs of oral or systemic disease, malformation, or injury, and the potential need for referral for diagnosis and treatment.

Diagnostic Imaging

Should be taken only for clinical reasons as determined by the patient's dentist. Should be of diagnostic quality and properly identified and dated. Is a part of the patient's clinical record and the original images should be retained by the dentist. Originals should not be used to fulfill requests made by patients or third-parties for copies of records.

Image Capture with Interpretation

D0210 **intraoral – complete series of radiographic images**

A radiographic survey of the whole mouth, usually consisting of 14-22 periapical and posterior bitewing images intended to display the crowns and roots of all teeth, periapical areas and alveolar bone.

D0220 **intraoral – periapical first radiographic image**

D0230 **intraoral – periapical each additional radiographic image**

D0240   intraoral – occlusal radiographic image

D0250   extraoral – first radiographic image

D0260   extraoral – each additional radiographic image

D0270   bitewing – single radiographic image

D0272   bitewings – two radiographic images

D0273   bitewings – three radiographic images

D0274   bitewings – four radiographic images

D0277   vertical bitewings – 7 to 8 radiographic images
This does not constitute a full mouth intraoral radiographic series.

D0290   posterior-anterior or lateral skull and facial bone survey radiographic image

D0310   sialography

D0320   temporomandibular joint arthrogram, including injection

D0321   other temporomandibular joint radiographic images, by report

D0322   tomographic survey

D0330   panoramic radiographic image

D0340   cephalometric radiographic image

▲ D0350   oral/facial photographic image obtained intraorally or extraorally

D0364   cone beam CT capture and interpretation with limited field of view – less than one whole jaw

D0365   cone beam CT capture and interpretation with field of view of one full dental arch – mandible

D0366   cone beam CT capture and interpretation with field of view of one full dental arch – maxilla, with or without cranium

● new procedure code   ▲ revision to a nomenclature or descriptor

D0367 cone beam CT capture and interpretation with field of view of both jaws; with or without cranium

D0368 cone beam CT capture and interpretation for TMJ series including two or more exposures

D0369 maxillofacial MRI capture and interpretation

D0370 maxillofacial ultrasound capture and interpretation

D0371 sialoendoscopy capture and interpretation

Image Capture Only

Interpretation and Report Performed by a Practitioner Not Associated With the Capture

D0380 cone beam CT image capture with limited field of view – less than one whole jaw

D0381 cone beam CT image capture with field of view of one full dental arch – mandible

D0382 cone beam CT image capture with field of view of one full dental arch – maxilla, with or without cranium

D0383 cone beam CT image capture with field of view of both jaws, with or without cranium

D0384 cone beam CT image capture for TMJ series including two or more exposures

D0385 maxillofacial MRI image capture

D0386 maxillofacial ultrasound image capture

Interpretation and Report Only

Image Capture Performed by a Practitioner Not Associated With Interpretation and Report

D0391 interpretation of diagnostic image by a practitioner not associated with capture of the image, including report

- **Post Processing of Image or Image Sets**

- **D0393 treatment simulation using 3D image volume**
  The use of 3D image volumes for simulation of treatment including, but not limited to, dental implant placement, orthognathic surgery and orthodontic tooth movement.

- **D0394 digital subtraction of two or more images or image volumes of the same modality**
  To demonstrate changes that have occurred over time.

- **D0395 fusion of two or more 3D image volumes of one or more modalities**

Tests and Examinations

D0415 collection of microorganisms for culture and sensitivity

D0416 viral culture
A diagnostic test to identify viral organisms, most often herpes virus.

D0417 collection and preparation of saliva sample for laboratory diagnostic testing

D0418 analysis of saliva sample
Chemical or biological analysis of saliva sample for diagnostic purposes.

D0421 genetic test for susceptibility to oral diseases
Sample collection for the purpose of certified laboratory analysis to detect specific genetic variations associated with increased susceptibility for oral diseases such as severe periodontal disease.

D0425 caries susceptibility tests
Not to be used for carious dentin staining.

D0431 adjunctive pre-diagnostic test that aids in detection of mucosal abnormalities including premalignant and malignant lesions, not to include cytology or biopsy procedures

D0460 pulp vitality tests
Includes multiple teeth and contra lateral comparison(s), as indicated.

● new procedure code   ▲ revision to a nomenclature or descriptor

D0470 diagnostic casts
    Also known as diagnostic models or study models.

Oral Pathology Laboratory (Use Codes D0472 – D0502)

These are procedures generally performed in a pathology laboratory and do not include the removal of the tissue sample from the patient. For removal of tissue sample, see codes D7285 and D7286.

D0472 accession of tissue, gross examination, preparation and transmission of written report
    To be used in reporting architecturally intact tissue obtained by invasive means.

D0473 accession of tissue, gross and microscopic examination, preparation and transmission of written report
    To be used in reporting architecturally intact tissue obtained by invasive means.

D0474 accession of tissue, gross and microscopic examination, including assessment of surgical margins for presence of disease, preparation and transmission of written report
    To be used in reporting architecturally intact tissue obtained by invasive means.

D0480 accession of exfoliative cytologic smears, microscopic examination, preparation and transmission of written report
    To be used in reporting disaggregated, non-transepithelial cell cytology sample via mild scraping of the oral mucosa.

D0486 laboratory accession of transepithelial cytologic sample, microscopic examination, preparation and transmission of written report
    Analysis, and written report of findings, of cytological sample of disaggregated transepithelial cells.

D0475 decalcification procedure
    Procedure in which hard tissue is processed in order to allow sectioning and subsequent microscopic examination.

D0476 **special stains for microorganisms**
Procedure in which additional stains are applied to biopsy or surgical specimen in order to identify microorganisms.

D0477 **special stains, not for microorganisms**
Procedure in which additional stains are applied to a biopsy or surgical specimen in order to identify such things as melanin, mucin, iron, glycogen, etc.

D0478 **immunohistochemical stains**
A procedure in which specific antibody based reagents are applied to tissue samples in order to facilitate diagnosis.

D0479 **tissue in-situ hybridization, including interpretation**
A procedure which allows for the identification of nucleic acids, DNA and RNA, in the tissue sample in order to aid in the diagnosis of microorganisms and tumors.

D0481 **electron microscopy – diagnostic**
An extreme high magnification diagnostic procedure that enables identification of cell components and microorganisms that are otherwise not identifiable under light microscopy.

D0482 **direct immunofluorescence**
A technique used to identify immunoreactants which are localized to the patient's skin or mucous membranes.

D0483 **indirect immunofluorescence**
A technique used to identify circulating immunoreactants.

D0484 **consultation on slides prepared elsewhere**
A service provided in which microscopic slides of a biopsy specimen prepared at another laboratory are evaluated to aid in the diagnosis of a difficult case or to offer a consultative opinion at the patient's request. The findings are delivered by written report.

D0485 **consultation, including preparation of slides from biopsy material supplied by referring source**
A service that requires the consulting pathologist to prepare the slides as well as render a written report. The slides are evaluated to aid in the diagnosis of a difficult case or to offer a consultative opinion at the patient's request.

D0502 **other oral pathology procedures, by report**

- D0601 **caries risk assessment and documentation, with a finding of low risk**
Using recognized assessment tools.

- D0602 **caries risk assessment and documentation, with a finding of moderate risk**
Using recognized assessment tools.

- D0603 **caries risk assessment and documentation, with a finding of high risk**
Using recognized assessment tools.

D0999 **unspecified diagnostic procedure, by report**
Used for procedure that is not adequately described by a code. Describe procedure.

D1000-D1999 II. Preventive

Dental Prophylaxis

D1110 prophylaxis – adult
Removal of plaque, calculus and stains from the tooth structures in the permanent and transitional dentition. It is intended to control local irritational factors.

D1120 prophylaxis – child
Removal of plaque, calculus and stains from the tooth structures in the primary and transitional dentition. It is intended to control local irritational factors.

Topical Fluoride Treatment (Office Procedure)

Prescription strength fluoride product designed solely for use in the dental office, delivered to the dentition under the direct supervision of a dental professional. Fluoride must be applied separately from prophylaxis paste.

D1206 topical application of fluoride varnish

D1208 topical application of fluoride

Other Preventive Services

D1310 nutritional counseling for control of dental disease
Counseling on food selection and dietary habits as a part of treatment and control of periodontal disease and caries.

D1320 tobacco counseling for the control and prevention of oral disease
Tobacco prevention and cessation services reduce patient risks of developing tobacco-related oral diseases and conditions and improves prognosis for certain dental therapies.

D1330 oral hygiene instructions
This may include instructions for home care. Examples include tooth brushing technique, flossing, and use of special oral hygiene aids.

D1351 sealant - per tooth
Mechanically and/or chemically prepared enamel surface sealed to prevent decay.

D1352 preventive resin restoration in a moderate to high caries risk patient – permanent tooth
Conservative restoration of an active cavitated lesion in a pit or fissure that does not extend into dentin; includes placement of a sealant in any radiating non-carious fissures or pits.

Space Maintenance (Passive Appliances)

Passive appliances are designed to prevent tooth movement.

D1510 space maintainer – fixed - unilateral

D1515 space maintainer – fixed - bilateral

D1520 space maintainer – removable – unilateral

D1525 space maintainer – removable – bilateral

D1550 re-cementation of space maintainer

D1555 removal of fixed space maintainer
Procedure delivered by dentist who did not originally place the appliance, or by the practice where the appliance was originally delivered to the patient.

- **D1999 unspecified preventive procedure, by report**

D2000–D2999 III. Restorative

Local anesthesia is usually considered to be part of Restorative procedures.

A one-surface posterior restoration is one in which the restoration involves only one of the five surface classifications (mesial, distal, occlusal, lingual, or facial, including buccal and labial).

A two-surface posterior restoration is one in which the restoration extends to two of the five surface classifications.

A three-surface posterior restoration is one in which the restoration extends to three of the five surface classifications.

A four-or-more surface posterior restoration is one in which the restoration extends to four or more of the five surface classifications.

A one-surface anterior proximal restoration is one in which neither the lingual nor the facial margins of the restoration extend beyond the line angle.

A two-surface anterior proximal restoration is one in which either the lingual or facial margin of the restoration extends beyond the line angle.

A three-surface anterior proximal restoration is one in which both the lingual and facial margins of the restorations extend beyond the line angle.

A four-or-more surface anterior restoration is one in which both the lingual and facial margins extend beyond the line angle and the incisal angle is involved. This restoration might also involve all four surfaces of an anterior tooth and not involve the incisal angle.

Amalgam Restorations (Including Polishing)

Tooth preparation, all adhesives (including amalgam bonding agents), liners and bases are included as part of the restoration. If pins are used, they should be reported separately (see D2951).

D2140   amalgam – one surface, primary or permanent

D2150   amalgam – two surfaces, primary or permanent

D2160   amalgam – three surfaces, primary or permanent

D2161   amalgam – four or more surfaces, primary or permanent

Resin-Based Composite Restorations – Direct

Resin-based composite refers to a broad category of materials including but not limited to composites. May include bonded composite, light-cured composite, etc. Tooth preparation, acid etching, adhesives (including resin bonding agents), liners and bases and curing are included as part of the restoration. Glass ionomers, when used as restorations, should be reported with these codes. If pins are used, they should be reported separately (see D2951).

D2330 resin-based composite – one surface, anterior

D2331 resin-based composite – two surfaces, anterior

D2332 resin-based composite – three surfaces, anterior

D2335 resin-based composite – four or more surfaces or involving incisal angle (anterior)
Incisal angle to be defined as one of the angles formed by the junction of the incisal and the mesial or distal surface of an anterior tooth.

D2390 resin-based composite crown, anterior
Full resin-based composite coverage of tooth.

D2391 resin-based composite – one surface, posterior
Used to restore a carious lesion into the dentin or a deeply eroded area into the dentin. Not a preventive procedure.

D2392 resin-based composite – two surfaces, posterior

D2393 resin-based composite – three surfaces, posterior

D2394 resin-based composite – four or more surfaces, posterior

Gold Foil Restorations

D2410 gold foil – one surface

D2420 gold foil – two surfaces

D2430 gold foil – three surfaces

● new procedure code ▲ revision to a nomenclature or descriptor

Inlay/Onlay Restorations

D2510 inlay – metallic – one surface

D2520 inlay – metallic – two surfaces

D2530 inlay – metallic – three or more surfaces

D2542 onlay – metallic – two surfaces

D2543 onlay – metallic – three surfaces

D2544 onlay – metallic – four or more surfaces

**Porcelain/ceramic inlays/onlays include all indirect ceramic
and porcelain type inlays/onlays.**

D2610 inlay – porcelain/ceramic – one surface

D2620 inlay – porcelain/ceramic – two surfaces

D2630 inlay – porcelain/ceramic – three or more surfaces

D2642 onlay – porcelain/ceramic – two surfaces

D2643 onlay – porcelain/ceramic – three surfaces

D2644 onlay – porcelain/ceramic – four or more surfaces

**Resin-based composite inlays/onlays must utilize
indirect technique.**

D2650 inlay – resin-based composite – one surface

D2651 inlay – resin-based composite – two surfaces

D2652 inlay – resin-based composite – three or more surfaces

D2662 onlay – resin-based composite – two surfaces

D2663 onlay – resin-based composite – three surfaces

D2664 onlay – resin-based composite – four or more surfaces

Crowns - Single Restorations Only

D2710 crown – resin-based composite (indirect)

D2712 crown – ¾ resin-based composite (indirect)
This code does not include facial veneers.

D2720 crown – resin with high noble metal

D2721 crown – resin with predominantly base metal

D2722 crown – resin with noble metal

D2740 crown – porcelain/ceramic substrate

D2750 crown – porcelain fused to high noble metal

D2751 crown – porcelain fused to predominantly base metal

D2752 crown – porcelain fused to noble metal

D2780 crown – ¾ cast high noble metal

D2781 crown – ¾ cast predominantly base metal

D2782 crown – ¾ cast noble metal

D2783 crown – ¾ porcelain/ceramic
This code does not include facial veneers.

D2790 crown – full cast high noble metal

D2791 crown – full cast predominantly base metal

D2792 crown – full cast noble metal

D2794 crown – titanium

D2799 provisional crown– further treatment or completion of diagnosis necessary prior to final impression
Not to be used as a temporary crown for a routine prosthetic restoration.

● new procedure code   ▲ revision to a nomenclature or descriptor

Other Restorative Services

D2990 resin infiltration of incipient smooth surface lesions
Placement of an infiltrating resin restoration for strengthening, stabilizing and/or limiting the progression of the lesion.

D2910 recement inlay, onlay, or partial coverage restoration

D2915 recement cast or prefabricated post and core

D2920 recement crown

• **D2921 reattachment of tooth fragment, incisal edge or cusp**

D2929 prefabricated porcelain/ceramic crown – primary tooth

D2930 prefabricated stainless steel crown – primary tooth

D2931 prefabricated stainless steel crown – permanent tooth

D2932 prefabricated resin crown

D2933 prefabricated stainless steel crown with resin window
Open-face stainless steel crown with aesthetic resin facing or veneer.

D2934 prefabricated esthetic coated stainless steel crown – primary tooth
Stainless steel primary crown with exterior esthetic coating.

D2940 protective restoration
Direct placement of a restorative material to protect tooth and/or tissue form. This procedure may be used to relieve pain, promote healing, or prevent further deterioration. Not to be used for endodontic access closure, or as a base or liner under restoration.

• **D2941 interim therapeutic restoration – primary dentition**
Placement of an adhesive restorative material following caries debridement by hand or other method for the management of early childhood caries. Not considered a definitive restoration.

- **D2949 restorative foundation for an indirect restoration**
  Placement of restorative material to yield a more ideal form, including elimination of undercuts.

▲ **D2950 core buildup, including any pins when required**
  Refers to building up of coronal structure when there is insufficient retention for a separate extracoronal restorative procedure. A core buildup is not a filler to eliminate any undercut, box form, or concave irregularity in a preparation.

D2951 pin retention – per tooth, in addition to restoration

D2952 post and core in addition to crown, indirectly fabricated
  Post and core are custom fabricated as a single unit.

D2953 each additional indirectly fabricated post – same tooth
  To be used with D2952.

D2954 prefabricated post and core in addition to crown
  Core is built around a prefabricated post. This procedure includes the core material.

D2955 post removal

D2957 each additional prefabricated post – same tooth
  To be used with D2954.

D2960 labial veneer (resin laminate) – chairside
  Refers to labial/facial direct resin bonded veneers.

D2961 labial veneer (resin laminate) – laboratory
  Refers to labial/facial indirect resin bonded veneers.

D2962 labial veneer (porcelain laminate) – laboratory
  Refers also to facial veneers that extend interproximally and/or cover the incisal edge. Porcelain/ceramic veneers presently include all ceramic and porcelain veneers.

D2970 temporary crown (fractured tooth)
  Usually a preformed artificial crown, which is fitted over a damaged tooth as an immediate protective device. This is not to be used as temporization during crown fabrication.

● new procedure code ▲ revision to a nomenclature or descriptor

D2971 additional procedures to construct new crown under existing partial denture framework
To be reported in addition to a crown code.

D2975 coping
A thin covering of the remaining portion of a tooth, usually fabricated of metal and devoid of anatomic contour. This is to be used as a definitive restoration.

D2980 crown repair necessitated by restorative material failure

D2981 inlay repair necessitated by restorative material failure

D2982 onlay repair necessitated by restorative material failure

D2983 veneer repair necessitated by restorative material failure

D2999 unspecified restorative procedure, by report
Use for procedure that is not adequately described by a code. Describe procedure.

D3000–D3999 IV. Endodontics

Local anesthesia is usually considered to be part of Endodontic procedures.

Pulp Capping

D3110 pulp cap – direct (excluding final restoration)
Procedure in which the exposed pulp is covered with a dressing or cement that protects the pulp and promotes healing and repair.

D3120 pulp cap – indirect (excluding final restoration)
Procedure in which the nearly exposed pulp is covered with a protective dressing to protect the pulp from additional injury and to promote healing and repair via formation of secondary dentin. This code is not to be used for bases and liners when all caries has been removed.

Pulpotomy

D3220 therapeutic pulpotomy (excluding final restoration) – removal of pulp coronal to the dentinocemental junction and application of medicament
Pulpotomy is the surgical removal of a portion of the pulp with the aim of maintaining the vitality of the remaining portion by means of an adequate dressing.

– To be performed on primary or permanent teeth.

– This is not to be construed as the first stage of root canal therapy.

– Not to be used for apexogenesis.

D3221 pulpal debridement, primary and permanent teeth
Pulpal debridement for the relief of acute pain prior to conventional root canal therapy. This procedure is not to be used when endodontic treatment is completed on the same day.

D3222 **partial pulpotomy for apexogenesis – permanent tooth with incomplete root development**
Removal of a portion of the pulp and application of a medicament with the aim of maintaining the vitality of the remaining portion to encourage continued physiological development and formation of the root. This procedure is not to be construed as the first stage of root canal therapy.

Endodontic Therapy on Primary Teeth

Endodontic therapy on primary teeth with succedaneous teeth and placement of resorbable filling. This includes pulpectomy, cleaning, and filling of canals with resorbable material.

D3230 **pulpal therapy (resorbable filling) – anterior, primary tooth (excluding final restoration)**
Primary incisors and cuspids.

D3240 **pulpal therapy (resorbable filling) – posterior, primary tooth (excluding final restoration)**
Primary first and second molars.

Endodontic Therapy (Including Treatment Plan, Clinical Procedures and Follow-Up Care)

Includes primary teeth without succedaneous teeth and permanent teeth. Complete root canal therapy; pulpectomy is part of root canal therapy.

Includes all appointments necessary to complete treatment; also includes intra-operative radiographs. Does not include diagnostic evaluation and necessary radiographs/diagnostic images.

D3310 **endodontic therapy, anterior tooth (excluding final restoration)**

D3320 **endodontic therapy, bicuspid tooth (excluding final restoration)**

D3330 **endodontic therapy, molar (excluding final restoration)**

● new procedure code   ▲ revision to a nomenclature or descriptor

D3331 **treatment of root canal obstruction; non-surgical access**
In lieu of surgery, the formation of a pathway to achieve an apical seal without surgical intervention because of a non-negotiable root canal blocked by foreign bodies, including but not limited to separated instruments, broken posts or calcification of 50% or more of the length of the tooth root.

D3332 **incomplete endodontic therapy; inoperable, unrestorable or fractured tooth**
Considerable time is necessary to determine diagnosis and/or provide initial treatment before the fracture makes the tooth unretainable.

D3333 **internal root repair of perforation defects**
Non-surgical seal of perforation caused by resorption and/or decay but not iatrogenic by provider filing claim.

Endodontic Retreatment

D3346 **retreatment of previous root canal therapy – anterior**

D3347 **retreatment of previous root canal therapy – bicuspid**

D3348 **retreatment of previous root canal therapy – molar**

▲ Apexification/Recalcification

▲ **D3351** **apexification/recalcification – initial visit (apical closure/ calcific repair of perforations, root resorption, pulp space disinfection, etc.)**
Includes opening tooth, preparation of canal spaces, first placement of medication and necessary radiographs. (This procedure may include first phase of complete root canal therapy.)

▲ **D3352** **apexification/recalcification – interim medication replacement**
For visits in which the intra-canal medication is replaced with new medication. Includes any necessary radiographs.

D3353 **apexification/recalcification – final visit (includes completed root canal therapy – apical closure/calcific repair of perforations, root resorption, etc.)**
Includes removal of intra-canal medication and procedures necessary to place final root canal filling material including necessary radiographs. (This procedure includes last phase of complete root canal therapy.)

• Pulpal Regeneration

- **D3355** **pulpal regeneration – initial visit**
Includes opening tooth, preparation of canal spaces, placement of medication.

- **D3356** **pulpal regeneration – interim medication replacement**

- **D3357** **pulpal regeneration – completion of treatment**
Does not include final restoration.

Apicoectomy/Periradicular Services

Periradicular surgery is a term used to describe surgery to the root surface (e.g., apicoectomy), repair of a root perforation or resorptive defect, exploratory curettage to look for root fractures, removal of extruded filling materials or instruments, removal of broken root fragments, sealing of accessory canals, etc. This does not include retrograde filling material placement.

▲ **D3410** **apicoectomy – anterior**
For surgery on root of anterior tooth. Does not include placement of retrograde filling material.

▲ **D3421** **apicoectomy – bicuspid (first root)**
For surgery on one root of a bicuspid. Does not include placement of retrograde filling material. If more than one root is treated, see D3426.

▲ **D3425** **apicoectomy – molar (first root)**
For surgery on one root of a molar tooth. Does not include placement of retrograde filling material. If more than one root is treated, see D3426.

● new procedure code   ▲ revision to a nomenclature or descriptor

▲ **D3426** **apicoectomy (each additional root)**
Typically used for bicuspids and molar surgeries when more than one root is treated during the same procedure. This does not include retrograde filling material placement.

• **D3427** **periradicular surgery without apicoectomy**

• **D3428** **bone graft in conjunction with periradicular surgery – per tooth, single site**
Includes non-autogenous graft material.

• **D3429** **bone graft in conjunction with periradicular surgery – each additional contiguous tooth in the same surgical site**
Includes non-autogenous graft material.

D3430 **retrograde filling – per root**
For placement of retrograde filling material during periradicular surgery procedures. If more than one filling is placed in one root report as D3999 and describe.

• **D3431** **biologic materials to aid in soft and osseous tissue regeneration in conjunction with periradicular surgery**

• **D3432** **guided tissue regeneration, resorbable barrier, per site, in conjunction with periradicular surgery**

D3450 **root amputation – per root**
Root resection of a multi-rooted tooth while leaving the crown. If the crown is sectioned, see D3920.

D3460 **endodontic endosseous implant**
Placement of implant material, which extends from a pulpal space into the bone beyond the end of the root.

D3470 **intentional reimplantation (including necessary splinting)**
For the intentional removal, inspection and treatment of the root and replacement of a tooth into its own socket. This does not include necessary retrograde filling material placement.

Other Endodontic Procedures

D3910 **surgical procedure for isolation of tooth with rubber dam**

D3920 **hemisection (including any root removal), not including root canal therapy**
Includes separation of a multi-rooted tooth into separate sections containing the root and the overlying portion of the crown. It may also include the removal of one or more of those sections.

D3950 **canal preparation and fitting of preformed dowel or post**
Should not be reported in conjunction with D2952, D2953, D2954 or D2957 by the same practitioner.

D3999 **unspecified endodontic procedure, by report**
Used for procedure that is not adequately described by a code. Describe procedure.

● new procedure code   ▲ revision to a nomenclature or descriptor

D4000-D4999   V. Periodontics

Local anesthesia is usually considered to be part of Periodontal procedures.

Surgical Services (Including Usual Postoperative Care)

Site: A term used to describe a single area, position, or locus. The word "site" is frequently used to indicate an area of soft tissue recession on a single tooth or an osseous defect adjacent to a single tooth; also used to indicate soft tissue defects and/or osseous defects in edentulous tooth positions.

- If two contiguous teeth have areas of soft tissue recession, each area of recession is a single site.

- If two contiguous teeth have adjacent but separate osseous defects, each defect is a single site.

- If two contiguous teeth have a communicating interproximal osseous defect, it should be considered a single site.

- All non-communicating osseous defects are single sites.

- All edentulous non-contiguous tooth positions are single sites.

- Depending on the dimensions of the defect, up to two contiguous edentulous tooth positions may be considered a single site.

Tooth Bounded Space: A space created by one or more missing teeth that has a tooth on each side.

D4210 **gingivectomy or gingivoplasty – four or more contiguous teeth or tooth bounded spaces per quadrant**
It is performed to eliminate suprabony pockets or to restore normal architecture when gingival enlargements or asymmetrical or unaesthetic topography is evident with normal bony configuration.

D4211 **gingivectomy or gingivoplasty – one to three contiguous teeth or tooth bounded spaces per quadrant**
It is performed to eliminate suprabony pockets or to restore normal architecture when gingival enlargements or asymmetrical or unaesthetic topography is evident with normal bony configuration.

D4212 **gingivectomy or gingivoplasty to allow access for restorative procedure, per tooth**

D4230 **anatomical crown exposure – four or more contiguous teeth per quadrant**
This procedure is utilized in an otherwise periodontally healthy area to remove enlarged gingival tissue and supporting bone (ostectomy) to provide an anatomically correct gingival relationship.

D4231 **anatomical crown exposure – one to three teeth per quadrant**
This procedure is utilized in an otherwise periodontally healthy area to remove enlarged gingival tissue and supporting bone (ostectomy) to provide an anatomically correct gingival relationship.

D4240 **gingival flap procedure, including root planing – four or more contiguous teeth or tooth bounded spaces per quadrant**
A soft tissue flap is reflected or resected to allow debridement of the root surface and the removal of granulation tissue. Osseous recontouring is not accomplished in conjunction with this procedure. May include open flap curettage, reverse bevel flap surgery, modified Kirkland flap procedure, and modified Widman surgery. This procedure is performed in the presence of moderate to deep probing depths, loss of attachment, need to maintain esthetics, need for increased access to the root surface and alveolar bone, or to determine the presence of a cracked tooth, fractured root, or external root resorption. Other procedures may be required concurrent to D4240 and should be reported separately using their own unique codes.

D4241 **gingival flap procedure, including root planing – one to three contiguous teeth or tooth bounded spaces per quadrant**
A soft tissue flap is reflected or resected to allow debridement of the root surface and the removal of granulation tissue. Osseous recontouring is not accomplished in conjunction with this procedure. May include open flap curettage, reverse bevel flap surgery, modified Kirkland flap procedure, and modified Widman surgery. This procedure is performed in the presence of moderate to deep probing depths, loss of attachment, need to maintain esthetics, need for increased access to the root surface and alveolar bone, or to determine the presence of a cracked tooth, fractured root, or external root resorption. Other procedures may be required concurrent to D4241 and should be reported separately using their own unique codes.

 © 2013 American Dental Association   ● new procedure code   ▲ revision to a nomenclature or descriptor

D4245 apically positioned flap

Procedure is used to preserve keratinized gingiva in conjunction with osseous resection and second stage implant procedure. Procedure may also be used to preserve keratinized/attached gingiva during surgical exposure of labially impacted teeth, and may be used during treatment of peri-implantitis.

D4249 clinical crown lengthening – hard tissue

This procedure is employed to allow restorative procedure or crown with little or no tooth structure exposed to the oral cavity. Crown lengthening requires reflection of a flap and is performed in a healthy periodontal environment, as opposed to osseous surgery, which is performed in the presence of periodontal disease. Where there are adjacent teeth, the flap design may involve a larger surgical area.

D4260 osseous surgery (including flap entry and closure) – four or more contiguous teeth or tooth bounded spaces per quadrant

This procedure modifies the bony support of the teeth by reshaping the alveolar process to achieve a more physiologic form. This must include the removal of supporting bone (ostectomy) and/or non-supporting bone (osteoplasty). Other procedures may be required concurrent to D4260 and should be reported using their own unique codes.

D4261 osseous surgery (including flap entry and closure) – one to three contiguous teeth or tooth bounded spaces per quadrant

This procedure modifies the bony support of the teeth by reshaping the alveolar process to achieve a more physiologic form. This must include the removal of supporting bone (ostectomy) and/or non-supporting bone (osteoplasty). Other procedures may be required concurrent to D4261 and should be reported using their own unique codes.

▲ **D4263 bone replacement graft – first site in quadrant**

This procedure involves the use of grafts to stimulate periodontal regeneration when the disease process has led to a deformity of the bone. This procedure does not include flap entry and closure, wound debridement, osseous contouring, or the placement of biologic materials to aid in osseous tissue regeneration or barrier membranes. Other separate procedures delivered concurrently are documented with their own codes.

▲ **D4264 bone replacement graft – each additional site in quadrant**
This procedure involves the use of grafts to stimulate periodontal regeneration when the disease process has led to a deformity of the bone. This procedure does not include flap entry and closure, wound debridement, osseous contouring, or the placement of biologic materials to aid in osseous tissue regeneration or barrier membranes. This procedure is performed concurrently with one or more bone replacement grafts to document the number of sites involved.

D4265 biologic materials to aid in soft and osseous tissue regeneration
Biologic materials may be used alone or with other regenerative substrates such as bone and barrier membranes, depending upon their formulation and the presentation of the periodontal defect. This procedure does not include surgical entry and closure, wound debridement, osseous contouring, or the placement of graft materials and/or barrier membranes. Other separate procedures may be required concurrent to D4265 and should be reported using their own unique codes.

D4266 guided tissue regeneration – resorbable barrier, per site
This procedure does not include flap entry and closure, or, when indicated, wound debridement, osseous contouring, bone replacement grafts, and placement of biologic materials to aid in osseous regeneration. This procedure can be used for periodontal and peri-implant defects.

D4267 guided tissue regeneration – non-resorbable barrier, per site (includes membrane removal)
This procedure does not include flap entry and closure, or, when indicated, wound debridement, osseous contouring, bone replacement grafts, and placement of biologic materials to aid in osseous regeneration. This procedure can be used for periodontal and peri-implant defects.

D4268 surgical revision procedure, per tooth
This procedure is to refine the results of a previously provided surgical procedure. This may require a surgical procedure to modify the irregular contours of hard or soft tissue. A mucoperiosteal flap may be elevated to allow access to reshape alveolar bone. The flaps are replaced or repositioned and sutured.

D4270 **pedicle soft tissue graft procedure**
A pedicle flap of gingiva can be raised from an edentulous ridge, adjacent teeth, or from the existing gingiva on the tooth and moved laterally or coronally to replace alveolar mucosa as marginal tissue. The procedure can be used to cover an exposed root or to eliminate a gingival defect if the root is not too prominent in the arch.

D4273 **subepithelial connective tissue graft procedures, per tooth**
This procedure is performed to create or augment gingiva, to obtain root coverage to eliminate sensitivity and to prevent root caries, to eliminate frenum pull, to extend the vestibular fornix, to augment collapsed ridges, to provide an adequate gingival interface with a restoration or to cover bone or ridge regeneration sites when adequate gingival tissues are not available for effective closure. There are two surgical sites. The recipient site utilizes a split thickness incision, retaining the overlying flap of gingiva and/ or mucosa. The connective tissue is dissected from the donor site leaving an epithelialized flap for closure. After the graft is placed on the recipient site, it is covered with the retained overlying flap.

D4274 **distal or proximal wedge procedure (when not performed in conjunction with surgical procedures in the same anatomical area)**
This procedure is performed in an edentulous area adjacent to a periodontally involved tooth. Gingival incisions are utilized to allow removal of a tissue wedge to gain access and correct the underlying osseous defect and to permit close flap adaptation.

D4275 **soft tissue allograft**
Procedure is performed to create or augment the gingiva, with or without root coverage. This may be used to eliminate the pull of the frena and muscle attachments, to extend the vestibular fornix, and correct localized gingival recession. There is no donor site.

D4276 **combined connective tissue and double pedicle graft, per tooth**
Advanced gingival recession often cannot be corrected with a single procedure. Combined tissue grafting procedures are needed to achieve the desired outcome.

D4277 **free soft tissue graft procedure (including donor site surgery), first tooth or edentulous tooth position in graft**

D4278 **free soft tissue graft procedure (including donor site surgery), each additional contiguous tooth or edentulous tooth position in same graft site**

Non-Surgical Periodontal Service

D4320 **provisional splinting – intracoronal**
This is an interim stabilization of mobile teeth. A variety of methods and appliances may be employed for this purpose. Identify the teeth involved.

D4321 **provisional splinting – extracoronal**
This is an interim stabilization of mobile teeth. A variety of methods and appliances may be employed for this purpose. Identify the teeth involved.

D4341 **periodontal scaling and root planing – four or more teeth per quadrant**
This procedure involves instrumentation of the crown and root surfaces of the teeth to remove plaque and calculus from these surfaces. It is indicated for patients with periodontal disease and is therapeutic, not prophylactic, in nature. Root planing is the definitive procedure designed for the removal of cementum and dentin that is rough, and/or permeated by calculus or contaminated with toxins or microorganisms. Some soft tissue removal occurs. This procedure may be used as a definitive treatment in some stages of periodontal disease and/or as a part of pre-surgical procedures in others.

D4342 **periodontal scaling and root planing – one to three teeth per quadrant**
This procedure involves instrumentation of the crown and root surfaces of the teeth to remove plaque and calculus from these surfaces. It is indicated for patients with periodontal disease and is therapeutic, not prophylactic, in nature. Root planing is the definitive procedure designed for the removal of cementum and dentin that is rough, and/or permeated by calculus or contaminated with toxins or microorganisms. Some soft tissue removal occurs. This procedure may be used as a definitive treatment in some stages of periodontal disease and/or as a part of pre-surgical procedures in others.

D4355 full mouth debridement to enable comprehensive evaluation and diagnosis

The gross removal of plaque and calculus that interfere with the ability of the dentist to perform a comprehensive oral evaluation. This preliminary procedure does not preclude the need for additional procedures.

D4381 localized delivery of antimicrobial agents via a controlled release vehicle into diseased crevicular tissue, per tooth

FDA approved subgingival delivery devices containing antimicrobial medication(s) are inserted into periodontal pockets to suppress the pathogenic microbiota. These devices slowly release the pharmacological agents so they can remain at the intended site of action in a therapeutic concentration for a sufficient length of time.

Other Periodontal Services

D4910 periodontal maintenance

This procedure is instituted following periodontal therapy and continues at varying intervals, determined by the clinical evaluation of the dentist, for the life of the dentition or any implant replacements. It includes removal of the bacterial plaque and calculus from supragingival and subgingival regions, site specific scaling and root planing where indicated, and polishing the teeth. If new or recurring periodontal disease appears, additional diagnostic and treatment procedures must be considered.

▲ **D4920 unscheduled dressing change (by someone other than treating dentist or their staff)**

• **D4921 gingival irrigation – per quadrant**

Irrigation of gingival pockets with medicinal agent. Not to be used to report use of mouth rinses or non-invasive chemical debridement.

D4999 unspecified periodontal procedure, by report

Use for procedure that is not adequately described by a code. Describe procedure.

D5000-D5899 VI. Prosthodontics (removable)

Local anesthesia is usually considered to be part of Removable Prosthodontic procedures.

Complete Dentures (Including Routine Post-Delivery Care)

D5110 **complete denture – maxillary**

D5120 **complete denture – mandibular**

D5130 **immediate denture – maxillary**
Includes limited follow-up care only; does not include required future rebasing/relining procedure(s) or a complete new denture.

D5140 **immediate denture – mandibular**
Includes limited follow-up care only; does not include required future rebasing/relining procedure(s) or a complete new denture.

Partial Dentures (Including Routine Post-Delivery Care)

D5211 **maxillary partial denture – resin base (including any conventional clasps, rests and teeth)**
Includes acrylic resin base denture with resin or wrought wire clasps.

D5212 **mandibular partial denture – resin base (including any conventional clasps, rests and teeth)**
Includes acrylic resin base denture with resin or wrought wire clasps.

D5213 **maxillary partial denture – cast metal framework with resin denture bases (including any conventional clasps, rests and teeth)**

D5214 **mandibular partial denture – cast metal framework with resin denture bases (including any conventional clasps, rests and teeth)**

D5225 **maxillary partial denture – flexible base (including any clasps, rests and teeth)**

D5226   mandibular partial denture – flexible base (including any clasps, rests and teeth)

D5281   removable unilateral partial denture – one piece cast metal (including clasps and teeth)

Adjustments to Dentures

D5410   adjust complete denture – maxillary

D5411   adjust complete denture – mandibular

D5421   adjust partial denture – maxillary

D5422   adjust partial denture – mandibular

Repairs to Complete Dentures

D5510   repair broken complete denture base

D5520   replace missing or broken teeth – complete denture (each tooth)

Repairs to Partial Dentures

D5610   repair resin denture base

D5620   repair cast framework

D5630   repair or replace broken clasp

D5640   replace broken teeth - per tooth

D5650   add tooth to existing partial denture

D5660   add clasp to existing partial denture

D5670   replace all teeth and acrylic on cast metal framework (maxillary)

D5671   replace all teeth and acrylic on cast metal framework (mandibular)

Denture Rebase Procedures

Rebase – process of refitting a denture by replacing the base material.

D5710 **rebase complete maxillary denture**

D5711 **rebase complete mandibular denture**

D5720 **rebase maxillary partial denture**

D5721 **rebase mandibular partial denture**

Denture Reline Procedures

Reline is the process of resurfacing the tissue side of a denture with new base material.

D5730 **reline complete maxillary denture (chairside)**

D5731 **reline complete mandibular denture (chairside)**

D5740 **reline maxillary partial denture (chairside)**

D5741 **reline mandibular partial denture (chairside)**

D5750 **reline complete maxillary denture (laboratory)**

D5751 **reline complete mandibular denture (laboratory)**

D5760 **reline maxillary partial denture (laboratory)**

D5761 **reline mandibular partial denture (laboratory)**

Interim Prosthesis

A provisional prosthesis designed for use over a limited period of time, after which it is to be replaced by a more definitive restoration.

D5810 **interim complete denture (maxillary)**

D5811 **interim complete denture (mandibular)**

D5820 interim partial denture (maxillary)
Includes any necessary clasps and rests.

D5821 interim partial denture (mandibular)
Includes any necessary clasps and rests.

Other Removable Prosthetic Services

D5850 tissue conditioning, maxillary
Treatment reline using materials designed to heal unhealthy ridges prior to more definitive final restoration.

D5851 tissue conditioning, mandibular
Treatment reline using materials designed to heal unhealthy ridges prior to more definitive final restoration.

D5862 precision attachment, by report
Each set of male and female components should be reported as one precision attachment. Describe the type of attachment used.

• **D5863 overdenture – complete maxillary**

• **D5864 overdenture – partial maxillary**

• **D5865 overdenture – complete mandibular**

• **D5866 overdenture – partial mandibular**

D5867 replacement of replaceable part of semi-precision or precision attachment (male or female component)

D5875 modification of removable prosthesis following implant surgery
The modification of existing removable prosthesis is sometimes necessary at the time of implant placement and bone graft surgery and is always necessary at the time of the placement of the healing caps. This code could also be used to report the modification of an existing prosthesis when the abutments are placed and retentive elements are placed into the removable prosthesis, thereby reducing the need for a new prosthesis.

D5899 unspecified removable prosthodontic procedure, by report
Use for a procedure that is not adequately described by a code. Describe procedure.

D5900–D5999 VII. Maxillofacial Prosthetics

D5911 facial moulage (sectional)
A sectional facial moulage impression is a procedure used to record the soft tissue contours of a portion of the face. Occasionally several separate sectional impressions are made, and then reassembled to provide a full facial contour cast. The impression is utilized to create a partial facial moulage and generally is not reusable.

D5912 facial moulage (complete)
Synonymous terminology: facial impression, face mask impression.

A complete facial moulage impression is a procedure used to record the soft tissue contours of the whole face. The impression is utilized to create a facial moulage and generally is not reusable.

D5913 nasal prosthesis
Synonymous terminology: artificial nose.

A removable prosthesis attached to the skin, which artificially restores part or all of the nose. Fabrication of a nasal prosthesis requires creation of an original mold. Additional prostheses usually can be made from the same mold, and assuming no further tissue changes occur, the same mold can be utilized for extended periods of time.

When a new prosthesis is made from the existing mold, this procedure is termed a nasal prosthesis replacement.

D5914 auricular prosthesis
Synonymous terminology: artificial ear, ear prosthesis.

A removable prosthesis, which artificially restores part or all of the natural ear. Usually, replacement prostheses can be made from the original mold if tissue bed changes have not occurred. Creation of an auricular prosthesis requires fabrication of a mold, from which additional prostheses usually can be made, as needed later (auricular prosthesis, replacement).

D5915 orbital prosthesis

A prosthesis, which artificially restores the eye, eyelids, and adjacent hard and soft tissue, lost as a result of trauma or surgery.

Fabrication of an orbital prosthesis requires creation of an original mold. Additional prostheses usually can be made from the same mold, and assuming no further tissue changes occur, the same mold can be utilized for extended periods of time.

When a new prosthesis is made from the existing mold, this procedure is termed an orbital prosthesis replacement.

D5916 ocular prosthesis

Synonymous terminology: artificial eye, glass eye.

A prosthesis, which artificially replaces an eye missing as a result of trauma, surgery or congenital absence. The prosthesis does not replace missing eyelids or adjacent skin, mucosa or muscle.

Ocular prostheses require semiannual or annual cleaning and polishing. Also, occasional revisions to re-adapt the prosthesis to the tissue bed may be necessary. Glass eyes are rarely made and cannot be re-adapted.

D5919 facial prosthesis

Synonymous terminology: prosthetic dressing.

A removable prosthesis, which artificially replaces a portion of the face, lost due to surgery, trauma or congenital absence.

Flexion of natural tissues may preclude adaptation and movement of the prosthesis to match the adjacent skin. Salivary leakage, when communicating with the oral cavity, adversely affects retention.

D5922 nasal septal prosthesis

Synonymous terminology: Septal plug, septal button.

Removable prosthesis to occlude (obturate) a hole within the nasal septal wall. Adverse chemical degradation in this moist environment may require frequent replacement. Silicone prostheses are occasionally subject to fungal invasion.

D5923 ocular prosthesis, interim

Synonymous terminology: Eye shell, shell, ocular conformer, conformer.

A temporary replacement generally made of clear acrylic resin for an eye lost due to surgery or trauma. No attempt is made to re-establish esthetics. Fabrication of an interim ocular prosthesis generally implies subsequent fabrication of an aesthetic ocular prosthesis.

D5924 cranial prosthesis

Synonymous terminology: Skull plate, cranioplasty prosthesis, cranial implant.

A biocompatible, permanently implanted replacement of a portion of the skull bones; an artificial replacement for a portion of the skull bone.

D5925 facial augmentation implant prosthesis

Synonymous terminology: facial implant.

An implantable biocompatible material generally onlayed upon an existing bony area beneath the skin tissue to fill in or collectively raise portions of the overlaying facial skin tissues to create acceptable contours.

Although some forms of pre-made surgical implants are commercially available, the facial augmentation is usually custom made for surgical implantation for each individual patient due to the irregular or extensive nature of the facial deficit.

D5926 nasal prosthesis, replacement

Synonymous terminology: replacement nose.

An artificial nose produced from a previously made mold. A replacement prosthesis does not require fabrication of a new mold. Generally, several prostheses can be made from the same mold assuming no changes occur in the tissue bed due to surgery or age related topographical variations.

D5927 auricular prosthesis, replacement

Synonymous terminology: replacement ear.

An artificial ear produced from a previously made mold. A replacement prosthesis does not require fabrication of a new mold. Generally, several prostheses can be made from the same mold assuming no changes occur in the tissue bed due to surgery or age related topographical variations.

D5928 orbital prosthesis, replacement

A replacement for a previously made orbital prosthesis. A replacement prosthesis does not require fabrication of a new mold. Generally, several prostheses can be made from the same mold assuming no changes occur in the tissue bed due to surgery or age related topographical variations.

D5929 facial prosthesis, replacement

A replacement facial prosthesis made from the original mold. A replacement prosthesis does not require fabrication of a new mold. Generally, several prostheses can be made from the same mold assuming no changes occur in the tissue bed due to further surgery or age related topographical variations.

D5931 obturator prosthesis, surgical

Synonymous terminology: Obturator, surgical stayplate, immediate temporary obturator.

A temporary prosthesis inserted during or immediately following surgical or traumatic loss of a portion or all of one or both maxillary bones and contiguous alveolar structures (e.g., gingival tissue, teeth).

Frequent revisions of surgical obturators are necessary during the ensuing healing phase (approximately six months). Some dentists prefer to replace many or all teeth removed by the surgical procedure in the surgical obturator, while others do not replace any teeth. Further surgical revisions may require fabrication of another surgical obturator (e.g., an initially planned small defect may be revised and greatly enlarged after the final pathology report indicates margins are not free of tumor).

D5932 obturator prosthesis, definitive

Synonymous terminology: obturator

A prosthesis, which artificially replaces part or all of the maxilla and associated teeth, lost due to surgery, trauma or congenital defects.

A definitive obturator is made when it is deemed that further tissue changes or recurrence of tumor are unlikely and a more permanent prosthetic rehabilitation can be achieved; it is intended for long-term use.

● new procedure code   ▲ revision to a nomenclature or descriptor

D5933 obturator prosthesis, modification
Synonymous terminology: adjustment, denture adjustment, temporary or office reline.

Revision or alteration of an existing obturator (surgical, interim, or definitive); possible modifications include relief of the denture base due to tissue compression, augmentation of the seal or peripheral areas to effect adequate sealing or separation between the nasal and oral cavities.

D5934 mandibular resection prosthesis with guide flange
Synonymous terminology: resection device, resection appliance.

A prosthesis which guides the remaining portion of the mandible, left after a partial resection, into a more normal relationship with the maxilla. This allows for some tooth-to-tooth or an improved tooth contact. It may also artificially replace missing teeth and thereby increase masticatory efficiency.

D5935 mandibular resection prosthesis without guide flange
A prosthesis which helps guide the partially resected mandible to a more normal relation with the maxilla allowing for increased tooth contact. It does not have a flange or ramp, however, to assist in directional closure. It may replace missing teeth and thereby increase masticatory efficiency.

Dentists who treat mandibulectomy patients may prefer to replace some, all or none of the teeth in the defect area. Frequently, the defect's margins preclude even partial replacement. Use of a guide (a mandibular resection prosthesis with a guide flange) may not be possible due to anatomical limitations or poor patient tolerance. Ramps, extended occlusal arrangements and irregular occlusal positioning relative to the denture foundation frequently preclude stability of the prostheses, and thus some prostheses are poorly tolerated under such adverse circumstances.

D5936 obturator prosthesis, interim

Synonymous terminology: immediate postoperative obturator.

A prosthesis which is made following completion of the initial healing after a surgical resection of a portion or all of one or both the maxillae; frequently many or all teeth in the defect area are replaced by this prosthesis. This prosthesis replaces the surgical obturator, which is usually inserted at, or immediately following the resection.

Generally, an interim obturator is made to facilitate closure of the resultant defect after initial healing has been completed. Unlike the surgical obturator, which usually is made prior to surgery and frequently revised in the operating room during surgery, the interim obturator is made when the defect margins are clearly defined and further surgical revisions are not planned. It is a provisional prosthesis, which may replace some or all lost teeth, and other lost bone and soft tissue structures. Also, it frequently must be revised (termed an obturator prosthesis modification) during subsequent dental procedures (e.g., restorations, gingival surgery) as well as to compensate for further tissue shrinkage before a definitive obturator prosthesis is made.

D5937 trismus appliance (not for TMD treatment)

Synonymous terminology: occlusal device for mandibular trismus, dynamic bite opener.

A prosthesis, which assists the patient in increasing their oral aperture width in order to eat as well as maintain oral hygiene.

Several versions and designs are possible, all intending to ease the severe lack of oral opening experienced by many patients immediately following extensive intraoral surgical procedures.

D5951 feeding aid

Synonymous terminology: feeding prosthesis.

A prosthesis, which maintains the right and left maxillary segments of an infant cleft palate patient in their proper orientation until surgery is performed to repair the cleft. It closes the oral-nasal cavity defect, thus enhancing sucking and swallowing.

Used on an interim basis, this prosthesis achieves separation of the oral and nasal cavities in infants born with wide clefts necessitating delayed closure. It is eliminated if surgical closure can be effected or, alternatively, with eruption of the deciduous dentition a pediatric speech aid may be made to facilitate closure of the defect.

● new procedure code   ▲ revision to a nomenclature or descriptor

D5952 **speech aid prosthesis, pediatric**
Synonymous terminology: nasopharyngeal obturator, speech appliance, obturator, cleft palate appliance, prosthetic speech aid, speech bulb.

A temporary or interim prosthesis used to close a defect in the hard and/or soft palate. It may replace tissue lost due to developmental or surgical alterations. It is necessary for the production of intelligible speech.

Normal lateral growth of the palatal bones necessitates occasional replacement of this prosthesis. Intermittent revisions of the obturator section can assist in maintenance of palatalpharyngeal closure (termed a speech aid prosthesis modification). Frequently, such prostheses are not fabricated before the deciduous dentition is fully erupted since clasp retention is often essential.

D5953 **speech aid prosthesis, adult**
Synonymous terminology: prosthetic speech appliance, speech aid, speech bulb.

A definitive prosthesis, which can improve speech in adult cleft palate patients either by obturating (sealing off) a palatal cleft or fistula, or occasionally by assisting an incompetent soft palate. Both mechanisms are necessary to achieve velopharyngeal competency.

Generally, this prosthesis is fabricated when no further growth is anticipated and the objective is to achieve long-term use. Hence, more precise materials and techniques are utilized. Occasionally such procedures are accomplished in conjunction with precision attachments in crown work undertaken on some or all maxillary teeth to achieve improved aesthetics.

D5954 **palatal augmentation prosthesis**
Synonymous terminology: superimposed prosthesis, maxillary glossectomy prosthesis, maxillary speech prosthesis, palatal drop prosthesis.

A removable prosthesis which alters the hard and/or soft palate's topographical form adjacent to the tongue.

D5955 palatal lift prosthesis, definitive

A prosthesis which elevates the soft palate superiorly and aids in restoration of soft palate functions which may be lost due to an acquired, congenital or developmental defect.

A definitive palatal lift is usually made for patients whose experience with an interim palatal lift has been successful, especially if surgical alterations are deemed unwarranted.

D5958 palatal lift prosthesis, interim

Synonymous terminology: diagnostic palatal lift.

A prosthesis which elevates and assists in restoring soft palate function which may be lost due to clefting, surgery, trauma or unknown paralysis. It is intended for interim use to determine its usefulness in achieving palatalpharyngeal competency or enhance swallowing reflexes.

This prosthesis is intended for interim use as a diagnostic aid to assess the level of possible improvement in speech intelligibility. Some clinicians believe use of a palatal lift on an interim basis may stimulate an otherwise flaccid soft palate to increase functional activity, subsequently lessening its need.

D5959 palatal lift prosthesis, modification

Synonymous terminology: revision of lift, adjustment.

Alterations in the adaptation, contour, form or function of an existing palatal lift necessitated due to tissue impingement, lack of function, poor clasp adaptation or the like.

D5960 speech aid prosthesis, modification

Synonymous terminology: adjustment, repair, revision.

Any revision of a pediatric or adult speech aid not necessitating its replacement.

Frequently, revisions of the obturating section of any speech aid are required to facilitate enhanced speech intelligibility. Such revisions or repairs do not require complete remaking of the prosthesis, thus extending its longevity.

D5982 surgical stent

Synonymous terminology: periodontal stent, skin graft stent, columellar stent.

Stents are utilized to apply pressure to soft tissues to facilitate healing and prevent cicatrization or collapse.

A surgical stent may be required in surgical and post-surgical revisions to achieve close approximation of tissues. Usually such materials as temporary or interim soft denture liners, gutta percha, or dental modeling impression compound may be used.

D5984 radiation shield

Synonymous terminology: radiation stent, tongue protector, lead shield.

An intraoral prosthesis designed to shield adjacent tissues from radiation during orthovoltage treatment of malignant lesions of the head and neck region.

D5985 radiation cone locator

Synonymous terminology: docking device, cone locator.

A prosthesis utilized to direct and reduplicate the path of radiation to an oral tumor during a split course of irradiation.

D5987 commissure splint

Synonymous terminology: lip splint.

A device placed between the lips, which assists in achieving increased opening between the lips. Use of such devices enhances opening where surgical, chemical or electrical alterations of the lips has resulted in severe restriction or contractures.

D5988 surgical splint

Synonymous terminology: Gunning splint, modified Gunning splint, labiolingual splint, fenestrated splint, Kingsley splint, cast metal splint.

Splints are designed to utilize existing teeth and/or alveolar processes as points of anchorage to assist in stabilization and immobilization of broken bones during healing. They are used to re-establish, as much as possible, normal occlusal relationships during the process of immobilization. Frequently, existing prostheses (e.g., a patient's complete dentures) can be modified to serve as surgical splints. Frequently, surgical splints have arch bars added to facilitate intermaxillary fixation. Rubber elastics may be used to assist in this process. Circummandibular eyelet hooks can be utilized for enhanced stabilization with wiring to adjacent bone.

D5992 adjust maxillofacial prosthetic appliance, by report

D5993 maintenance and cleaning of a maxillofacial prosthesis (extra or intraoral) other than required adjustments, by report

Maintenance and cleaning of a maxillofacial prosthesis.

• Carriers

D5983 radiation carrier

Synonymous terminology: radiotherapy prosthesis, carrier prosthesis, radiation applicator, radium carrier, intracavity carrier, intracavity applicator.

A device used to administer radiation to confined areas by means of capsules, beads or needles of radiation emitting materials such as radium or cesium. Its function is to hold the radiation source securely in the same location during the entire period of treatment.

Radiation oncologists occasionally request these devices to achieve close approximation and controlled application of radiation to a tumor deemed amiable to eradication.

D5986 fluoride gel carrier

Synonymous terminology: fluoride applicator.

A prosthesis, which covers the teeth in either dental arch and is used to apply topical fluoride in close proximity to tooth enamel and dentin for several minutes daily.

● new procedure code   ▲ revision to a nomenclature or descriptor

▲ **D5991** **vesiculobullous disease medicament carrier**
A custom fabricated carrier that covers the teeth and alveolar mucosa, or alveolar mucosa alone, and is used to deliver prescription medicaments for treatment of immunologically mediated vesiculobullous diseases.

● **D5994** **periodontal medicament carrier with peripheral seal – laboratory processed**
A custom fabricated, laboratory processed carrier that covers the teeth and alveolar mucosa. Used as a vehicle to deliver prescribed medicaments for sustained contact with the gingiva, alveolar mucosa, and into the periodontal sulcus or pocket.

D5999 **unspecified maxillofacial prosthesis, by report**
Used for procedure that is not adequately described by a code. Describe procedure.

D6000–D6199   VIII. Implant Services

Local anesthesia is usually considered to be part of Implant Services procedures.

Pre-Surgical Services

D6190   radiographic/surgical implant index, by report
An appliance, designed to relate osteotomy or fixture position to existing anatomic structures, to be utilized during radiographic exposure for treatment planning and/or during osteotomy creation for fixture installation.

Surgical Services

Report surgical implant procedure using codes in this section.

▲ **D6010   surgical placement of implant body: endosteal implant**

● **D6011   second stage implant surgery**
Surgical access to an implant body for placement of a healing cap or to enable placement of an abutment.

D6012   surgical placement of interim implant body for transitional prosthesis: endosteal implant
Includes removal during later therapy to accommodate the definitive restoration, which may include placement of other implants.

● **D6013   surgical placement of mini implant**

D6040   surgical placement: eposteal implant
An eposteal (subperiosteal) framework of a biocompatible material designed and fabricated to fit on the surface of the bone of the mandible or maxilla with permucosal extensions which provide support and attachment of a prosthesis. This may be a complete arch or unilateral appliance. Eposteal implants rest upon the bone and under the periosteum.

D6050 surgical placement: transosteal implant
A transosteal (transosseous) biocompatible device with threaded posts penetrating both the superior and inferior cortical bone plates of the mandibular symphysis and exiting through the permucosa providing support and attachment for a dental prosthesis. Transosteal implants are placed completely through the bone and into the oral cavity from extraoral or intraoral.

D6100 implant removal, by report
This procedure involves the surgical removal of an implant. Describe procedure.

D6101 debridement of a periimplant defect and surface cleaning of exposed implant surfaces, including flap entry and closure

D6102 debridement and osseous contouring of a periimplant defect; includes surface cleaning of exposed implant surfaces and flap entry and closure

D6103 bone graft for repair of periimplant defect – not including flap entry and closure or, when indicated, placement of a barrier membrane or biologic materials to aid in osseous regeneration

D6104 bone graft at time of implant placement
Placement of a barrier membrane, or biologic materials to aid in osseous regeneration are reported separately.

Implant Supported Prosthetics

Supporting Structures

D6055 connecting bar – implant supported or abutment supported
Utilized to stabilize and anchor a prosthesis.

D6056 prefabricated abutment – includes modification and placement
Modification of a prefabricated abutment may be necessary.

D6057 custom fabricated abutment – includes placement
Created by a laboratory process, specific for an individual application.

D6051 interim abutment
Includes placement and removal. A healing cap is not an interim abutment.

● new procedure code   ▲ revision to a nomenclature or descriptor

- **D6052 semi-precision attachment abutment**
  Includes placement of keeper assembly.

Implant/Abutment Supported Removable Dentures

D6053 implant/abutment supported removable denture for completely edentulous arch

D6054 implant/abutment supported removable denture for partially edentulous arch

Implant/Abutment Supported Fixed Dentures (Hybrid Prosthesis)

D6078 implant/abutment supported fixed denture for completely edentulous arch
A prosthesis that is retained, supported and stabilized by implants or abutments placed on implants but does not have specific relationships between implant positions and replacement teeth; may be screw retained or cemented; commonly referred to as a "hybrid prosthesis."

D6079 implant/abutment supported fixed denture for partially edentulous arch
A prosthesis that is retained, supported and stabilized by implants or abutments placed on implants but does not have specific relationship between implant positions and replacement teeth; may be screw retained or cemented; commonly referred to as a "hybrid prosthesis".

Single Crowns, Abutment Supported

D6058 abutment supported porcelain/ceramic crown
A single crown restoration that is retained, supported and stabilized by an abutment on an implant; may be screw retained or cemented.

D6059 abutment supported porcelain fused to metal crown (high noble metal)
A single metal-ceramic crown restoration that is retained, supported and stabilized by an abutment on an implant; may be screw retained or cemented.

D6060 abutment supported porcelain fused to metal crown (predominantly base metal)
A single metal-ceramic crown restoration that is retained, supported and stabilized by an abutment on an implant; may be screw retained or cemented.

D6061 abutment supported porcelain fused to metal crown (noble metal)
A single metal-ceramic crown restoration that is retained, supported and stabilized by an abutment on an implant; may be screw retained or cemented.

D6062 abutment supported cast metal crown (high noble metal)
A single cast metal crown restoration that is retained, supported and stabilized by an abutment on an implant; may be screw retained or cemented.

D6063 abutment supported cast metal crown (predominantly base metal)
A single cast metal crown restoration that is retained, supported and stabilized by an abutment on an implant; may be screw retained or cemented.

D6064 abutment supported cast metal crown (noble metal)
A single cast metal crown restoration that is retained, supported and stabilized by an abutment on an implant; may be screw retained or cemented.

D6094 abutment supported crown (titanium)
A single crown restoration that is retained, supported and stabilized by an abutment on an implant. May be cast or milled and is screw retained or cemented.

Single Crowns, Implant Supported

D6065 implant supported porcelain/ceramic crown
A single crown restoration that is retained, supported and stabilized by an implant; may be screw retained or cemented.

● new procedure code   ▲ revision to a nomenclature or descriptor

D6066 **implant supported porcelain fused to metal crown (titanium, titanium alloy, high noble metal)**
A single metal-ceramic crown restoration that is retained, supported and stabilized by an implant; may be screw retained or cemented.

D6067 **implant supported metal crown (titanium, titanium alloy, high noble metal)**
A single cast metal or milled crown restoration that is retained, supported and stabilized by an implant; may be screw retained or cemented.

Fixed Partial Denture, Abutment Supported

D6068 **abutment supported retainer for porcelain/ceramic FPD**
A ceramic retainer for a fixed partial denture that gains retention, support and stability from an abutment on an implant; may be screw retained or cemented.

D6069 **abutment supported retainer for porcelain fused to metal FPD (high noble metal)**
A metal-ceramic retainer for a fixed partial denture that gains retention, support and stability from an abutment on an implant; may be screw retained or cemented.

D6070 **abutment supported retainer for porcelain fused to metal FPD (predominantly base metal)**
A metal-ceramic retainer for a fixed partial denture that gains retention, support and stability from an abutment on an implant; may be screw retained or cemented.

D6071 **abutment supported retainer for porcelain fused to metal FPD (noble metal)**
A metal-ceramic retainer for a fixed partial denture that gains retention, support and stability from an abutment on an implant; may be screw retained or cemented.

D6072 **abutment supported retainer for cast metal FPD (high noble metal)**
A cast metal retainer for a fixed partial denture that gains retention, support and stability from an abutment on an implant; may be screw retained or cemented.

D6073 **abutment supported retainer for cast metal FPD (predominantly base metal)**
A cast metal retainer for a fixed partial denture that gains retention, support and stability from an abutment on an implant; may be screw retained or cemented.

D6074 **abutment supported retainer for cast metal FPD (noble metal)**
A cast metal retainer for a fixed partial denture that gains retention, support and stability from an abutment on an implant; may be screw retained or cemented.

D6194 **abutment supported retainer crown for FPD titanium)**
A retainer for a fixed partial denture that gains retention, support and stability from an abutment on an implant. May be cast or milled and is screw retained or cemented.

Fixed Partial Denture, Implant Supported

D6075 **implant supported retainer for ceramic FPD**
A ceramic retainer for a fixed partial denture that gains retention, support and stability from an implant; may be screw retained or cemented.

D6076 **implant supported retainer for porcelain fused to metal FPD (titanium, titanium alloy, or high noble metal)**
A metal-ceramic retainer for a fixed partial denture that gains retention, support and stability from an implant; may be screw retained or cemented.

D6077 **implant supported retainer for cast metal FPD (titanium, titanium alloy, or high noble metal)**
A cast metal retainer for a fixed partial denture that gains retention, support and stability from an implant; may be screw retained or cemented.

 © 2013 American Dental Association   ● new procedure code   ▲ revision to a nomenclature or descriptor

Other Implant Services

▲ **D6080 implant maintenance procedures when prostheses are removed and reinserted, including cleansing of prostheses and abutments**
This procedure includes active debriding of the implant(s) and examination of all aspects of the implant system(s), including the occlusion and stability of the superstructure. The patient is also instructed in thorough daily cleansing of the implant(s). This is not a per implant code, and is indicated for implant supported fixed prostheses.

D6090 repair implant supported prosthesis, by report
This procedure involves the repair or replacement of any part of the implant supported prosthesis.

D6095 repair implant abutment, by report
This procedure involves the repair or replacement of any part of the implant abutment.

D6091 replacement of semi-precision or precision attachment (male or female component) of implant/abutment supported prosthesis, per attachment
This procedure applies to the replaceable male or female component of the attachment.

D6092 recement implant/abutment supported crown

D6093 recement implant/abutment supported fixed partial denture

D6199 unspecified implant procedure, by report
Use for procedure that is not adequately described by a code. Describe procedure.

D6200-D6999 IX. Prosthodontics, fixed

Each retainer and each pontic constitutes a unit in a fixed partial denture.

Local anesthesia is usually considered to be part of Fixed Prosthodontic procedures.

The term "fixed partial denture" replaces the words "bridge" and "bridgework" throughout this section.

Fixed partial denture prosthetic procedures include routine temporary prosthetics. When indicated, interim or provisional codes should be reported separately.

Fixed Partial Denture Pontics

D6205 pontic – indirect resin based composite
Not to be used as a temporary or provisional prosthesis.

D6210 pontic – cast high noble metal

D6211 pontic – cast predominantly base metal

D6212 pontic – cast noble metal

D6214 pontic – titanium

D6240 pontic – porcelain fused to high noble metal

D6241 pontic – porcelain fused to predominantly base metal

D6242 pontic – porcelain fused to noble metal

D6245 pontic – porcelain/ceramic

D6250 pontic – resin with high noble metal

D6251 pontic – resin with predominantly base metal

D6252 pontic – resin with noble metal

D6253 provisional pontic– further treatment or completion of diagnosis necessary prior to final impression
Not to be used as a temporary pontic for routine prosthetic fixed partial dentures.

Fixed Partial Denture Retainers — Inlays/Onlays

D6545 retainer — cast metal for resin bonded fixed prosthesis

D6548 retainer — porcelain/ceramic for resin bonded fixed prosthesis

D6600 inlay — porcelain/ceramic, two surfaces

D6601 inlay — porcelain/ceramic, three or more surfaces

D6602 inlay — cast high noble metal, two surfaces

D6603 inlay — cast high noble metal, three or more surfaces

D6604 inlay — cast predominantly base metal, two surfaces

D6605 inlay — cast predominantly base metal, three or more surfaces

D6606 inlay — cast noble metal, two surfaces

D6607 inlay — cast noble metal, three or more surfaces

D6624 inlay — titanium

D6608 onlay — porcelain/ceramic, two surfaces

D6609 onlay — porcelain/ceramic, three or more surfaces

D6610 onlay — cast high noble metal, two surfaces

D6611 onlay — cast high noble metal, three or more surfaces

D6612 onlay — cast predominantly base metal, two surfaces

D6613 onlay — cast predominantly base metal, three or more surfaces

D6614 onlay — cast noble metal, two surfaces

D6615 onlay — cast noble metal, three or more surfaces

D6634 onlay — titanium

 © 2013 American Dental Association ● new procedure code ▲ revision to a nomenclature or descriptor

Fixed Partial Denture Retainers – Crowns

D6710 **crown – indirect resin based composite**
Not to be used as a temporary or provisional prosthesis.

D6720 **crown – resin with high noble metal**

D6721 **crown – resin with predominantly base metal**

D6722 **crown – resin with noble metal**

D6740 **crown – porcelain/ceramic**

D6750 **crown – porcelain fused to high noble metal**

D6751 **crown – porcelain fused to predominantly base metal**

D6752 **crown – porcelain fused to noble metal**

D6780 **crown – ¾ cast high noble metal**

D6781 **crown – ¾ cast predominantly base metal**

D6782 **crown – ¾ cast noble metal**

D6783 **crown – ¾ porcelain/ceramic**

D6790 **crown – full cast high noble metal**

D6791 **crown – full cast predominantly base metal**

D6792 **crown – full cast noble metal**

D6794 **crown – titanium**

D6793 **provisional retainer crown– further treatment or completion of diagnosis necessary prior to final impression**
Not to be used as a temporary retainer crown for routine prosthetic fixed partial dentures.

Other Fixed Partial Denture Services

D6920 connector bar
A device attached to fixed partial denture retainer or coping which serves to stabilize and anchor a removable overdenture prosthesis.

D6930 recement fixed partial denture

D6940 stress breaker
A non-rigid connector.

D6950 precision attachment
A male and female pair constitutes one precision attachment, and is separate from the prosthesis.

D6975 coping
To be used as a definitive restoration when coping is an integral part of a fixed prosthesis.

D6980 fixed partial denture repair necessitated by restorative material failure

D6985 pediatric partial denture, fixed
This prosthesis is used primarily for aesthetic purposes.

D6999 unspecified fixed prosthodontic procedure, by report
Used for procedure that is not adequately described by a code. Describe procedure.

● new procedure code   ▲ revision to a nomenclature or descriptor

D7000-D7999   X. Oral and Maxillofacial Surgery

Local anesthesia is usually considered to be part of Oral and Maxillofacial Surgical procedures.

For dental benefit reporting purposes a quadrant is defined as four or more contiguous teeth and/or teeth spaces distal to the midline.

Extractions (Includes Local Anesthesia, Suturing, If Needed, and Routine Postoperative Care)

D7111   extraction, coronal remnants – deciduous tooth
Removal of soft tissue-retained coronal remnants.

D7140   extraction, erupted tooth or exposed root (elevation and/or forceps removal)
Includes routine removal of tooth structure, minor smoothing of socket bone, and closure, as necessary.

Surgical Extractions (Includes Local Anesthesia, Suturing, If Needed, and Routine Postoperative Care)

D7210   surgical removal of erupted tooth requiring removal of bone and/or sectioning of tooth, and including elevation of mucoperiosteal flap if indicated
Includes related cutting of gingiva and bone, removal of tooth structure, minor smoothing of socket bone and closure.

D7220   removal of impacted tooth – soft tissue
Occlusal surface of tooth covered by soft tissue; requires mucoperiosteal flap elevation.

D7230   removal of impacted tooth – partially bony
Part of crown covered by bone; requires mucoperiosteal flap elevation and bone removal.

D7240   removal of impacted tooth – completely bony
Most or all of crown covered by bone; requires mucoperiosteal flap elevation and bone removal.

D7241 **removal of impacted tooth – completely bony, with unusual surgical complications**
Most or all of crown covered by bone; unusually difficult or complicated due to factors such as nerve dissection required, separate closure of maxillary sinus required or aberrant tooth position.

D7250 **surgical removal of residual tooth roots (cutting procedure)**
Includes cutting of soft tissue and bone, removal of tooth structure, and closure.

D7251 **coronectomy – intentional partial tooth removal**
Intentional partial tooth removal is performed when a neurovascular complication is likely if the entire impacted tooth is removed.

Other Surgical Procedures

D7260 **oroantral fistula closure**
Excision of fistulous tract between maxillary sinus and oral cavity and closure by advancement flap.

D7261 **primary closure of a sinus perforation**
Subsequent to surgical removal of tooth, exposure of sinus requiring repair, or immediate closure of oroantral or oralnasal communication in absence of fistulous tract.

D7270 **tooth reimplantation and/or stabilization of accidentally evulsed or displaced tooth**
Includes splinting and/or stabilization.

D7272 **tooth transplantation (includes reimplantation from one site to another and splinting and/or stabilization)**

D7280 **surgical access of an unerupted tooth**
An incision is made and the tissue is reflected and bone removed as necessary to expose the crown of an impacted tooth not intended to be extracted.

D7282 **mobilization of erupted or malpositioned tooth to aid eruption**
To move/luxate teeth to eliminate ankylosis; not in conjunction with an extraction.

D7283 **placement of device to facilitate eruption of impacted tooth**
Placement of an orthodontic bracket, band or other device on an unerupted tooth, after its exposure, to aid in its eruption. Report the surgical exposure separately using D7280.

D7285 **biopsy of oral tissue – hard (bone, tooth)**
For removal of specimen only. This code involves biopsy of osseous lesions and is not used for apicoectomy/periradicular surgery.

D7286 **biopsy of oral tissue – soft**
For surgical removal of an architecturally intact specimen only. This code is not used at the same time as codes for apicoectomy/periradicular curettage.

D7287 **exfoliative cytological sample collection**
For collection of non-transepithelial cytology sample via mild scraping of the oral mucosa.

D7288 **brush biopsy – transepithelial sample collection**
For collection of oral disaggregated transepithelial cells via rotational brushing of the oral mucosa.

D7290 **surgical repositioning of teeth**
Grafting procedure(s) is/are additional.

D7291 **transseptal fiberotomy/supra crestal fiberotomy, by report**
The supraosseous connective tissue attachment is surgically severed around the involved teeth. Where there are adjacent teeth, the transseptal fiberotomy of a single tooth will involve a minimum of three teeth. Since the incisions are within the gingival sulcus and tissue and the root surface is not instrumented, this procedure heals by the reunion of connective tissue with the root surface on which viable periodontal tissue is present (reattachment).

D7292 **surgical placement: temporary anchorage device [screw retained plate] requiring surgical flap**
Insertion of a temporary skeletal anchorage device that is attached to the bone by screws and requires a surgical flap. Includes device removal.

D7293 **surgical placement: temporary anchorage device requiring surgical flap**
Insertion of a device for temporary skeletal anchorage when a surgical flap is required. Includes device removal.

D7294 **surgical placement: temporary anchorage device without surgical flap**
Insertion of a device for temporary skeletal anchorage when a surgical flap is not required. Includes device removal.

D7295 **harvest of bone for use in autogenous grafting procedure**
Reported in addition to those autogenous graft placement procedures that do not include harvesting of bone.

Alveoloplasty - Surgical Preparation of Ridge

D7310 **alveoloplasty in conjunction with extractions – four or more teeth or tooth spaces, per quadrant**
The alveoloplasty is distinct (separate procedure) from extractions and/or surgical extractions. Usually in preparation for a prosthesis or other treatments such as radiation therapy and transplant surgery.

D7311 **alveoloplasty in conjunction with extractions – one to three teeth or tooth spaces, per quadrant**
The alveoloplasty is distinct (separate procedure) from extractions and/or surgical extractions. Usually in preparation for a prosthesis or other treatments such as radiation therapy and transplant surgery.

D7320 **alveoloplasty not in conjunction with extractions – four or more teeth or tooth spaces, per quadrant**
No extractions performed in an edentulous area. See D7310 if teeth are being extracted concurrently with the alveoloplasty. Usually in preparation for a prosthesis or other treatments such as radiation therapy and transplant surgery.

D7321 **alveoloplasty not in conjunction with extractions – one to three teeth or tooth spaces, per quadrant**
No extractions performed in an edentulous area. See D7311 if teeth are being extracted concurrently with the alveoloplasty. Usually in preparation for a prosthesis or other treatments such as radiation therapy and transplant surgery.

Vestibuloplasty

Any of a series of surgical procedures designed to increase relative alveolar ridge height.

D7340 vestibuloplasty – ridge extension (secondary epithelialization)

D7350 vestibuloplasty – ridge extension (including soft tissue grafts, muscle reattachment, revision of soft tissue attachment and management of hypertrophied and hyperplastic tissue)

Surgical Excision of Soft Tissue Lesions

Includes non-odontogenic cysts.

D7410 excision of benign lesion up to 1.25 cm

D7411 excision of benign lesion greater than 1.25 cm

D7412 excision of benign lesion, complicated
Requires extensive undermining with advancement or rotational flap closure.

D7413 excision of malignant lesion up to 1.25 cm

D7414 excision of malignant lesion greater than 1.25 cm

D7415 excision of malignant lesion, complicated
Requires extensive undermining with advancement or rotational flap closure

D7465 destruction of lesion(s) by physical or chemical method, by report
Examples include using cryo, laser or electro surgery.

Surgical Excision of Intra-Osseous Lesions

D7440 excision of malignant tumor – lesion diameter up to 1.25 cm

D7441 excision of malignant tumor – lesion diameter greater than 1.25 cm

D7450 removal of benign odontogenic cyst or tumor – lesion diameter up to 1.25 cm

D7451 removal of benign odontogenic cyst or tumor – lesion diameter greater than 1.25 cm

D7460 removal of benign nonodontogenic cyst or tumor – lesion diameter up to 1.25 cm

D7461 removal of benign nonodontogenic cyst or tumor – lesion diameter greater than 1.25 cm

Excision of Bone Tissue

D7471 removal of lateral exostosis (maxilla or mandible)

D7472 removal of torus palatinus

D7473 removal of torus mandibularis

D7485 surgical reduction of osseous tuberosity

D7490 radical resection of maxilla or mandible
Partial resection of maxilla or mandible; removal of lesion and defect with margin of normal appearing bone. Reconstruction and bone grafts should be reported separately.

Surgical Incision

D7510 incision and drainage of abscess – intraoral soft tissue
Involves incision through mucosa, including periodontal origins.

D7511 incision and drainage of abscess – intraoral soft tissue – complicated (includes drainage of multiple fascial spaces)
Incision is made intraorally and dissection is extended into adjacent fascial space(s) to provide adequate drainage of abscess/cellulitis.

D7520 incision and drainage of abscess – extraoral soft tissue
Involves incision through skin.

D7521 **incision and drainage of abscess – extraoral soft tissue – complicated (includes drainage of multiple fascial spaces)**
Incision is made extraorally and dissection is extended into adjacent fascial space(s) to provide adequate drainage of abscess/cellulitis.

D7530 **removal of foreign body from mucosa, skin, or subcutaneous alveolar tissue**

D7540 **removal of reaction producing foreign bodies, musculoskeletal system**
May include, but is not limited to, removal of splinters, pieces of wire, etc., from muscle and/or bone.

D7550 **partial ostectomy/sequestrectomy for removal of non-vital bone**
Removal of loose or sloughed-off dead bone caused by infection or reduced blood supply.

D7560 **maxillary sinusotomy for removal of tooth fragment or foreign body**

Treatment of Fractures - Simple

D7610 **maxilla – open reduction (teeth immobilized, if present)**
Teeth may be wired, banded or splinted together to prevent movement. Surgical incision required for interosseous fixation.

D7620 **maxilla – closed reduction (teeth immobilized, if present)**
No incision required to reduce fracture. See D7610 if interosseous fixation is applied.

D7630 **mandible – open reduction (teeth immobilized, if present)**
Teeth may be wired, banded or splinted together to prevent movement. Surgical incision required to reduce fracture.

D7640 **mandible – closed reduction (teeth immobilized, if present)**
No incision required to reduce fracture. See D7630 if interosseous fixation is applied.

D7650 **malar and/or zygomatic arch – open reduction**

D7660 **malar and/or zygomatic arch – closed reduction**

D7670 alveolus – closed reduction, may include stabilization of teeth
Teeth may be wired, banded or splinted together to prevent movement.

D7671 alveolus – open reduction, may include stabilization of teeth
Teeth may be wired, banded or splinted together to prevent movement.

D7680 facial bones – complicated reduction with fixation and multiple surgical approaches
Facial bones include upper and lower jaw, cheek, and bones around eyes, nose, and ears.

Treatment of Fractures - Compound

D7710 maxilla – open reduction
Surgical incision required to reduce fracture.

D7720 maxilla – closed reduction

D7730 mandible – open reduction
Surgical incision required to reduce fracture.

D7740 mandible – closed reduction

D7750 malar and/or zygomatic arch – open reduction
Surgical incision required to reduce fracture.

D7760 malar and/or zygomatic arch – closed reduction

D7770 alveolus - open reduction stabilization of teeth
Fractured bone(s) are exposed to mouth or outside the face. Surgical incision required to reduce fracture.

D7771 alveolus, closed reduction stabilization of teeth
Fractured bone(s) are exposed to mouth or outside the face.

D7780 facial bones – complicated reduction with fixation and multiple surgical approaches
Surgical incision required to reduce fracture. Facial bones include upper and lower jaw, cheek, and bones around eyes, nose, and ears.

Reduction of Dislocation and Management of Other Temporomandibular Joint Dysfunctions

Procedures that are an integral part of a primary procedure should not be reported separately.

D7810 open reduction of dislocation
Access to TMJ via surgical opening.

D7820 closed reduction of dislocation
Joint manipulated into place; no surgical exposure.

D7830 manipulation under anesthesia
Usually done under general anesthesia or intravenous sedation.

D7840 condylectomy
Surgical removal of all or portion of the mandibular condyle (separate procedure).

D7850 surgical discectomy, with/without implant
Excision of the intra-articular disc of a joint.

D7852 disc repair
Repositioning and/or sculpting of disc; repair of perforated posterior attachment.

D7854 synovectomy
Excision of a portion or all of the synovial membrane of a joint.

D7856 myotomy
Cutting of muscle for therapeutic purposes (separate procedure).

D7858 joint reconstruction
Reconstruction of osseous components including or excluding soft tissues of the joint with autogenous, homologous, or alloplastic materials.

D7860 arthrotomy
Cutting into joint (separate procedure).

D7865 arthroplasty
Reduction of osseous components of the joint to create a pseudoarthrosis or eliminate an irregular remodeling pattern (osteophytes).

D7870 arthrocentesis
Withdrawal of fluid from a joint space by aspiration.

D7871 non-arthroscopic lysis and lavage
Inflow and outflow catheters are placed into the joint space. The joint is lavaged and manipulated as indicated in an effort to release minor adhesions and synovial vacuum phenomenon as well as to remove inflammation products from the joint space.

D7872 arthroscopy – diagnosis, with or without biopsy

D7873 arthroscopy – surgical: lavage and lysis of adhesions
Removal of adhesions using the arthroscope and lavage of the joint cavities.

D7874 arthroscopy – surgical: disc repositioning and stabilization
Repositioning and stabilization of disc using arthroscopic techniques.

D7875 arthroscopy – surgical: synovectomy
Removal of inflamed and hyperplastic synovium (partial/complete) via an arthroscopic technique.

D7876 arthroscopy – surgical: discectomy
Removal of disc and remodeled posterior attachment via the arthroscope.

D7877 arthroscopy – surgical: debridement
Removal of pathologic hard and/or soft tissue using the arthroscope.

D7880 occlusal orthotic device, by report
Presently includes splints provided for treatment of temporomandibular joint dysfunction.

D7899 unspecified TMD therapy, by report
Used for procedure that is not adequately described by a code. Describe procedure.

Repair of Traumatic Wounds

Excludes closure of surgical incisions.

D7910 suture of recent small wounds up to 5 cm

Complicated Suturing (Reconstruction Requiring Delicate Handling of Tissues and Wide Undermining for Meticulous Closure)

Excludes closure of surgical incisions.

D7911 **complicated suture – up to 5 cm**

D7912 **complicated suture – greater than 5 cm**

Other Repair Procedures

D7920 **skin graft (identify defect covered, location and type of graft)**

D7921 **collection and application of autologous blood concentrate product**

D7940 **osteoplasty – for orthognathic deformities**
Reconstruction of jaws for correction of congenital, developmental or acquired traumatic or surgical deformity.

D7941 **osteotomy – mandibular rami**

D7943 **osteotomy – mandibular rami with bone graft; includes obtaining the graft**

D7944 **osteotomy – segmented or subapical**
Report by range of tooth numbers within segment.

D7945 **osteotomy – body of mandible**
Surgical section of lower jaw. This includes the surgical exposure, bone cut, fixation, routine wound closure and normal post-operative follow-up care.

D7946 **LeFort I (maxilla – total)**
Surgical section of the upper jaw. This includes the surgical exposure, bone cuts, downfracture, repositioning, fixation, routine wound closure and normal post-operative follow-up care.

D7947 LeFort I (maxilla – segmented)
When reporting a surgically assisted palatal expansion without downfracture, this code would entail a reduced service and should be "by report."

D7948 LeFort II or LeFort III (osteoplasty of facial bones for midface hypoplasia or retrusion) – without bone graft
Surgical section of upper jaw. This includes the surgical exposure, bone cuts, downfracture, segmentation of maxilla, repositioning, fixation, routine wound closure and normal post-operative follow-up care.

D7949 LeFort II or LeFort III – with bone graft
Includes obtaining autografts.

▲ **D7950 osseous, osteoperiosteal, or cartilage graft of the mandible or maxilla – autogenous or nonautogenous, by report**
This procedure is for ridge augmentation or reconstruction to increase height, width and/or volume of residual alveolar ridge. It includes obtaining graft material. Placement of a barrier membrane, if used, should be reported separately.

D7951 sinus augmentation with bone or bone substitutes via a lateral open approach
The augmentation of the sinus cavity to increase alveolar height for reconstruction of edentulous portions of the maxilla. This procedure is performed via a lateral open approach. This includes obtaining the bone or bone substitutes. Placement of a barrier membrane if used should be reported separately.

D7952 sinus augmentation via a vertical approach
The augmentation of the sinus to increase alveolar height by vertical access through the ridge crest by raising the floor of the sinus and grafting as necessary. This includes obtaining the bone or bone substitutes.

▲ **D7953 bone replacement graft for ridge preservation – per site**
Graft is placed in an extraction or implant removal site at the time of the extraction or removal to preserve ridge integrity (e.g., clinically indicated in preparation for implant reconstruction or where alveolar contour is critical to planned prosthetic reconstruction). Does not include obtaining graft material. Membrane, if used should be reported separately.

▲ **D7955 repair of maxillofacial soft and/or hard tissue defect**
Reconstruction of surgical, traumatic, or congenital defects of the
facial bones, including the mandible, may utilize graft materials in
conjunction with soft tissue procedures to repair and restore the
facial bones to form and function. This does not include obtaining the
graft and these procedures may require multiple surgical approaches.
This procedure does not include edentulous maxilla and mandibular
reconstruction for prosthetic considerations.

**D7960 frenulectomy – also known as frenectomy or frenotomy –
separate procedure not incidental to another procedure**
Surgical removal or release of mucosal and muscle elements of a
buccal, labial or lingual frenum that is associated with a pathological
condition, or interferes with proper oral development or treatment.

D7963 frenuloplasty
Excision of frenum with accompanying excision or repositioning
of aberrant muscle and z-plasty or other local flap closure.

D7970 excision of hyperplastic tissue – per arch

D7971 excision of pericoronal gingiva
Surgical removal of inflammatory or hypertrophied tissues
surrounding partially erupted/impacted teeth.

D7972 surgical reduction of fibrous tuberosity

D7980 sialolithotomy
Surgical procedure by which a stone within a salivary gland or its
duct is removed, either intraorally or extraorally.

D7981 excision of salivary gland, by report

D7982 sialodochoplasty
Surgical procedure for the repair of a defect and/or restoration
of a portion of a salivary gland duct.

D7983 closure of salivary fistula
Surgical closure of an opening between a salivary duct and/or gland
and the cutaneous surface, or an opening into the oral cavity through
other than the normal anatomic pathway.

D7990 **emergency tracheotomy**
Surgical formation of a tracheal opening usually below the cricoid cartilage to allow for respiratory exchange.

D7991 **coronoidectomy**
Surgical removal of the coronoid process of the mandible.

D7995 **synthetic graft – mandible or facial bones, by report**
Includes allogenic material.

D7996 **implant-mandible for augmentation purposes (excluding alveolar ridge), by report**

D7997 **appliance removal (not by dentist who placed appliance), includes removal of archbar**

D7998 **intraoral placement of a fixation device not in conjunction with a fracture**
The placement of intermaxillary fixation appliance for documented medically accepted treatments not in association with fractures.

D7999 **unspecified oral surgery procedure, by report**
Used for procedure that is not adequately described by a code. Describe procedure.

 © 2013 American Dental Association   ● new procedure code   ▲ revision to a nomenclature or descriptor

D8000–D8999 XI. Orthodontics

Dentition

Primary Dentition: Teeth developed and erupted first in order of time.

Transitional Dentition: The final phase of the transition from primary to adult teeth, in which the deciduous molars and canines are in the process of shedding and the permanent successors are emerging.

Adolescent Dentition: The dentition that is present after the normal loss of primary teeth and prior to cessation of growth that would affect orthodontic treatment.

Adult Dentition: The dentition that is present after the cessation of growth that would affect orthodontic treatment.

All of the following orthodontic treatment codes may be used more than once for the treatment of a particular patient depending on the particular circumstance. A patient may require more than one interceptive procedure or more than one limited procedure depending on their particular problem.

▲ Limited Orthodontic Treatment

Orthodontic treatment with a limited objective, not necessarily involving the entire dentition. It may be directed at the only existing problem, or at only one aspect of a larger problem in which a decision is made to defer or forego more comprehensive therapy.

D8010 **limited orthodontic treatment of the primary dentition**

D8020 **limited orthodontic treatment of the transitional dentition**

D8030 **limited orthodontic treatment of the adolescent dentition**

D8040 **limited orthodontic treatment of the adult dentition**

▲ Interceptive Orthodontic Treatment

Interceptive orthodontics is an extension of preventive orthodontics that may include localized tooth movement. Such treatment may occur in the primary or transitional dentition and may include such procedures as the redirection of ectopically erupting teeth, correction of dental crossbite or recovery of space loss where overall space is inadequate. When initiated during the incipient stages of a developing problem, interceptive orthodontics may reduce the severity of the malformation and mitigate its cause. Complicating factors such as skeletal disharmonies, overall space deficiency, or other conditions may require subsequent comprehensive therapy.

D8050 interceptive orthodontic treatment of the primary dentition

D8060 interceptive orthodontic treatment of the transitional dentition

▲ Comprehensive Orthodontic Treatment

Comprehensive orthodontic care includes a coordinated diagnosis and treatment leading to the improvement of a patient's craniofacial dysfunction and/or dentofacial deformity which may include anatomical, functional and/or aesthetic relationships. Treatment may utilize fixed and/or removable orthodontic appliances and may also include functional and/or orthopedic appliances in growing and non-growing patients. Adjunctive procedures to facilitate care may be required. Comprehensive orthodontics may incorporate treatment phases focusing on specific objectives at various stages of dentofacial development.

D8070 comprehensive orthodontic treatment of the transitional dentition

D8080 comprehensive orthodontic treatment of the adolescent dentition

D8090 comprehensive orthodontic treatment of the adult dentition

 © 2013 American Dental Association   ● new procedure code   ▲ revision to a nomenclature or descriptor

Minor Treatment to Control Harmful Habits

D8210 removable appliance therapy
Removable indicates patient can remove; includes appliances for thumb sucking and tongue thrusting.

D8220 fixed appliance therapy
Fixed indicates patient cannot remove appliance; includes appliances for thumb sucking and tongue thrusting.

Other Orthodontic Services

D8660 pre-orthodontic treatment visit

D8670 periodic orthodontic treatment visit (as part of contract)

D8680 orthodontic retention (removal of appliances, construction and placement of retainer(s))

D8690 orthodontic treatment (alternative billing to a contract fee)
Services provided by dentist other than original treating dentist. A method of payment between the provider and responsible party for services that reflect an open-ended fee arrangement.

D8691 repair of orthodontic appliance
Does not include bracket and standard fixed orthodontic appliances. It does include functional appliances and palatal expanders.

D8692 replacement of lost or broken retainer

▲ **D8693 rebonding or recementing of fixed retainers**

● **D8694 repair of fixed retainers, includes reattachment**

D8999 unspecified orthodontic procedure, by report
Used for procedure that is not adequately described by a code. Describe procedure.

D9000-D9999 XII. Adjunctive General Services

Unclassified Treatment

D9110 palliative (emergency) treatment of dental pain - minor procedure
This is typically reported on a "per visit" basis for emergency treatment of dental pain.

D9120 fixed partial denture sectioning
Separation of one or more connections between abutments and/or pontics when some portion of a fixed prosthesis is to remain intact and serviceable following sectioning and extraction or other treatment. Includes all recontouring and polishing of retained portions.

Anesthesia

D9210 local anesthesia not in conjunction with operative or surgical procedures

D9211 regional block anesthesia

D9212 trigeminal division block anesthesia

D9215 local anesthesia in conjunction with operative or surgical procedures

D9220 deep sedation/general anesthesia – first 30 minutes
Anesthesia time begins when the doctor administering the anesthetic agent initiates the appropriate anesthesia and non-invasive monitoring protocol and remains in continuous attendance of the patient. Anesthesia services are considered completed when the patient may be safely left under the observation of trained personnel and the doctor may safely leave the room to attend to other patients or duties.

The level of anesthesia is determined by the anesthesia provider's documentation of the anesthetic's effects upon the central nervous system and not dependent upon the route of administration.

D9221 **deep sedation/general anesthesia – each additional 15 minutes**
Anesthesia time begins when the doctor administering the anesthetic agent initiates the appropriate anesthesia and non-invasive monitoring protocol and remains in continuous attendance of the patient. Anesthesia services are considered completed when the patient may be safely left under the observation of trained personnel and the doctor may safely leave the room to attend to other patients or duties.

The level of anesthesia is determined by the anesthesia provider's documentation of the anesthetic's effects upon the central nervous system and not dependent upon the route of administration.

D9230 **inhalation of nitrous oxide/analgesia, anxiolysis**

D9241 **intravenous conscious sedation/analgesia – first 30 minutes**
Anesthesia time begins when the doctor administering the anesthetic agent initiates the appropriate anesthesia and non-invasive monitoring protocol and remains in continuous attendance of the patient. Anesthesia services are considered completed when the patient may be safely left under the observation of trained personnel and the doctor may safely leave the room to attend to other patients or duties.

The level of anesthesia is determined by the anesthesia provider's documentation of the anesthetic's effects upon the central nervous system and not dependent upon the route of administration.

D9242 **intravenous conscious sedation/analgesia – each additional 15 minutes**
Anesthesia time begins when the doctor administering the anesthetic agent initiates the appropriate anesthesia and non-invasive monitoring protocol and remains in continuous attendance of the patient. Anesthesia services are considered completed when the patient may be safely left under the observation of trained personnel and the doctor may safely leave the room to attend to other patients or duties.

The level of anesthesia is determined by the anesthesia provider's documentation of the anesthetic's effects upon the central nervous system and not dependent upon the route of administration.

D9248 **non-intravenous conscious sedation**
A medically controlled state of depressed consciousness while maintaining the patient's airway, protective reflexes and the ability to respond to stimulation or verbal commands. It includes non-intravenous administration of sedative and/or analgesic agent(s) and appropriate monitoring.

The level of anesthesia is determined by the anesthesia provider's documentation of the anesthetic's effects upon the central nervous system and not dependent upon the route of administration.

Professional Consultation

D9310 **consultation – diagnostic service provided by dentist or physician other than requesting dentist or physician**
A patient encounter with a practitioner whose opinion or advice regarding evaluation and/or management of a specific problem; may be requested by another practitioner or appropriate source. The consultation includes an oral evaluation. The consulted practitioner may initiate diagnostic and/or therapeutic services.

Professional Visits

D9410 **house/extended care facility call**
Includes visits to nursing homes, long-term care facilities, hospice sites, institutions, etc. Report in addition to reporting appropriate code numbers for actual services performed.

D9420 **hospital or ambulatory surgical center call**
Care provided outside the dentist's office to a patient who is in a hospital or ambulatory surgical center. Services delivered to the patient on the date of service are documented separately using the applicable procedure codes.

D9430 **office visit for observation (during regularly scheduled hours) – no other services performed**

D9440 **office visit – after regularly scheduled hours**

D9450 **case presentation, detailed and extensive treatment planning**
Established patient. Not performed on same day as evaluation.

Drugs

D9610 therapeutic parenteral drug, single administration
Includes single administration of antibiotics, steroids, anti-inflammatory drugs, or other therapeutic medications. This code should not be used to report administration of sedative, anesthetic or reversal agents.

D9612 therapeutic parenteral drugs, two or more administrations, different medications
Includes multiple administrations of antibiotics, steroids, anti-inflammatory drugs or other therapeutic medications. This code should not be used to report administration of sedatives, anesthetic or reversal agents.

This code should be reported when two or more different medications are necessary and should not be reported in addition to code D9610 on the same date.

D9630 other drugs and/or medicaments, by report
Includes, but is not limited to oral antibiotics, oral analgesics, and topical fluoride dispensed in the office for home use; does not include writing prescriptions.

Miscellaneous Services

D9910 application of desensitizing medicament
Includes in-office treatment for root sensitivity. Typically reported on a "per visit" basis for application of topical fluoride. This code is not to be used for bases, liners or adhesives used under restorations.

D9911 application of desensitizing resin for cervical and/or root surface, per tooth
Typically reported on a "per tooth" basis for application of adhesive resins. This code is not to be used for bases, liners, or adhesives used under restorations.

D9920 behavior management, by report
May be reported in addition to treatment provided. Should be reported in 15-minute increments.

D9930 **treatment of complications (post-surgical) – unusual circumstances, by report**

For example, treatment of a dry socket following extraction or removal of bony sequestrum.

D9940 **occlusal guard, by report**

Removable dental appliances, which are designed to minimize the effects of bruxism (grinding) and other occlusal factors.

D9941 **fabrication of athletic mouthguard**

D9942 **repair and/or reline of occlusal guard**

D9950 **occlusion analysis - mounted case**

Includes, but is not limited to, facebow, interocclusal records tracings, and diagnostic wax-up; for diagnostic casts, see D0470.

D9951 **occlusal adjustment – limited**

May also be known as equilibration; reshaping the occlusal surfaces of teeth to create harmonious contact relationships between the maxillary and mandibular teeth. Presently includes discing/odontoplasty/enamoplasty. Typically reported on a "per visit" basis. This should not be reported when the procedure only involves bite adjustment in the routine post-delivery care for a direct/indirect restoration or fixed/removable prosthodontics.

D9952 **occlusal adjustment – complete**

Occlusal adjustment may require several appointments of varying length, and sedation may be necessary to attain adequate relaxation of the musculature. Study casts mounted on an articulating instrument may be utilized for analysis of occlusal disharmony. It is designed to achieve functional relationships and masticatory efficiency in conjunction with restorative treatment, orthodontics, orthognathic surgery, or jaw trauma when indicated. Occlusal adjustment enhances the healing potential of tissues affected by the lesions of occlusal trauma.

D9970 **enamel microabrasion**

The removal of discolored surface enamel defects resulting from altered mineralization or decalcification of the superficial enamel layer. Submit per treatment visit.

D9971 odontoplasty 1-2 teeth; includes removal of enamel projections

D9972 external bleaching – per arch – performed in office

D9973 external bleaching – per tooth

D9974 internal bleaching – per tooth

D9975 external bleaching for home application, per arch; includes materials and fabrication of custom trays

● **D9985** sales tax

D9999 unspecified adjunctive procedure, by report
Used for procedure that is not adequately described by a code. Describe procedure.

2 Changes to the CDT Code

ADA American Dental Association®

America's leading advocate for oral health

Changes to the CDT Code

This version of the CDT Code is effective January 1, 2014 through December 31, 2014. All changes are illustrated in this section, with text additions <u>underlined in blue ink</u> and deleted text ~~stricken through in red ink~~. There are:

- 29 new code entries

- 18 revised code entries

- 4 deleted code entries, and

- 7 actions affecting subcategories or their descriptors.

As noted in the preface, the CDT Code is divided into twelve Categories of Service <u>only</u> for the purpose of organization. Each category begins at the top of a right-hand page in this section.

© 2013 American Dental Association

D0100-D0999   I. Diagnostic

Additions

One (1) Sub-subcategory of service

Post Processing of Image or Image Sets

Six (6) procedure codes

- **D0393** **treatment simulation using 3D image volume**
  The use of 3D image volumes for simulation of treatment including, but not limited to, dental implant placement, orthognathic surgery and orthodontic tooth movement.

- **D0394** **digital subtraction of two or more images or image volumes of the same modality**
  To demonstrate changes that have occurred over time.

- **D0395** **fusion of two or more 3D image volumes of one or more modalities**

- **D0601** **caries risk assessment and documentation, with a finding of low risk**
  Using recognized assessment tools.

- **D0602** **caries risk assessment and documentation, with a finding of moderate risk**
  Using recognized assessment tools.

- **D0603** **caries risk assessment and documentation, with a finding of high risk**
  Using recognized assessment tools.

Revisions
One (1) procedure code

▲ **D0350** **oral/facial photographic image** <u>obtained intraorally or extraorally</u>
~~This includes photographic images, including those obtained by intraoral and extraoral cameras, excluding radiographic images. These photographic images should be a part of the patient's clinical record.~~

Deletions
One (1) procedure code

~~**D0363**~~ ~~**cone beam three-dimensional image reconstruction using existing data, includes multiple images**~~

 © 2013 American Dental Association

D1000-D1999 II. Preventive

Additions
One (1) procedure code

- **D1999** **unspecified preventive procedure, by report**

Revisions
None

Deletions
None

D2000-D2999   III. Restorative

Additions
Three (3) procedure codes

- **D2921** **reattachment of tooth fragment, incisal edge or cusp**

- **D2941** **interim therapeutic restoration – primary dentition**
  Placement of an adhesive restorative material following caries debridement by hand or other method for the management of early childhood caries. Not considered a definitive restoration.

- **D2949** **restorative foundation for an indirect restoration**
  Placement of restorative material to yield a more ideal form, including elimination of undercuts.

Revisions
One (1) procedure code

▲ **D2950** **core buildup, including any pins when required**
  Refers to building up of coronal structure anatomical crown when restorative crown will be placed, whether or not pins are used. A material is placed in the tooth preparation for a crown when there is insufficient tooth strength and retention for the crown a separate extracoronal restorative procedure. A core buildup is not This should not be reported when the procedure only involves a filler to eliminate any undercut, box form, or concave irregularity in the a preparation.

Deletions
None

D3000–D3999   IV. Endodontics

Additions
One (1) Sub-subcategory of service

Pulpal Regeneration

Eight (8) procedure codes

- **D3355** **pulpal regeneration – initial visit**
  Includes opening tooth, preparation of canal spaces, placement of medication.

- **D3356** **pulpal regeneration – interim medication replacement**

- **D3357** **pulpal regeneration – completion of treatment**
  Does not include final restoration.

- **D3427** **periradicular surgery without apicoectomy**

- **D3428** **bone graft in conjunction with periradicular surgery – per tooth, single site**
  Includes non-autogenous graft material.

- **D3429** **bone graft in conjunction with periradicular surgery – each additional contiguous tooth in the same surgical site**
  Includes non-autogenous graft material.

- **D3431** **biologic materials to aid in soft and osseous tissue regeneration in conjunction with periradicular surgery**

- **D3432** **guided tissue regeneration, resorbable barrier, per site, in conjunction with periradicular surgery**

Revisions
One (1) Sub-subcategory of service

Apexification/Recalcification ~~and Pulpal Regeneration Procedures~~

Six (6) procedure codes

▲ **D3351** **apexification/recalcification~~/pulpal regeneration~~ – initial visit (apical closure/calcific repair of perforations, root resorption, pulp space disinfection, etc.)**
Includes opening tooth, preparation of canal spaces, first placement of medication and necessary radiographs. (This procedure may include first phase of complete root canal therapy.)

▲ **D3352** **apexification/recalcification~~/pulpal regeneration~~ – interim medication replacement**
For visits in which the intra-canal medication is replaced with new medication. Includes any necessary radiographs.

▲ **D3410** **apicoectomy~~/periradicular surgery~~ – anterior**
For surgery on root of anterior tooth. Does not include placement of retrograde filling material.

▲ **D3421** **apicoectomy~~/periradicular surgery~~ – bicuspid (first root)**
For surgery on one root of a bicuspid. Does not include placement of retrograde filling material. If more than one root is treated, see D3426.

▲ **D3425** **apicoectomy~~/periradicular surgery~~ – molar (first root)**
For surgery on one root of a molar tooth. Does not include placement of retrograde filling material. If more than one root is treated, see D3426.

▲ **D3426** **apicoectomy~~/periradicular surgery~~ – each additional root**
Typically used for bicuspids and molar surgeries when more than one root is treated during the same procedure. This does not include retrograde filling material placement.

Deletions

One (1) procedure code

~~**D3354**~~ ~~**pulpal regeneration – (completion of regenerative treatment in an immature permanent tooth with a necrotic pulp); does not include final restoration**~~
~~Includes removal of intra-canal medication and procedures necessary to regenerate continued root development and necessary radiographs. This procedure includes placement of a seal at the coronal portion of the root canal system. Conventional root canal treatment is not performed.~~

D4000-D4999   V. Periodontics

Additions
One (1) procedure code

- **D4921   gingival irrigation – per quadrant**
  Irrigation of gingival pockets with medicinal agent. Not to be used to report use of mouth rinses or non-invasive chemical debridement.

Revisions
Three (3) procedure codes

▲ **D4263   bone replacement graft – first site in quadrant**
This procedure involves the use of ~~osseous autografts, osseous allografts, or non-osseous~~ grafts to stimulate periodontal regeneration when the disease process has led to a deformity of the bone. This procedure does not include flap entry and closure, wound debridement, osseous contouring, or the placement of biologic materials to aid in osseous tissue regeneration or barrier membranes. Other separate procedures delivered concurrently are documented with ~~may be required concurrent to D4263 and should be reported using~~ their own ~~unique~~ codes.

▲ **D4264   bone replacement graft – each additional site in quadrant**
This procedure involves the use of ~~osseous autografts, osseous allografts, or non-osseous~~ grafts to stimulate periodontal regeneration when the disease process has led to a deformity of the bone. This procedure does not include flap entry and closure, wound debridement, osseous contouring, or the placement of biologic materials to aid in osseous tissue regeneration or barrier membranes. This procedure ~~code~~ is ~~used if~~ performed concurrently with one or more bone replacement grafts to document ~~D4263 and allows reporting of~~ the ~~exact~~ number of sites involved.

▲ **D4920   unscheduled dressing change (by someone other than treating dentist or their staff)**

Deletions
None

D5000-D5899 VI. Prosthodontics (removable)

Additions
Four (4) procedure codes

- **D5863** **overdenture – complete maxillary**

- **D5864** **overdenture – partial maxillary**

- **D5865** **overdenture – complete mandibular**

- **D5866** **overdenture – partial mandibular**

Revisions
None

Deletions
Two (2) procedure codes

D5860 **overdenture – complete, by report**
Describe and document procedures as performed. Other separate procedures may be required concurrent to D5860.

D5861 **overdenture – partial, by report**
Describe and document procedures as performed. Other separate procedures may be required concurrent to D5861.

D5900-D5999   VII. Maxillofacial Prosthetics

Additions
One (1) Subcategory of service

Carriers

One (1) procedure code

- **D5994** **periodontal medicament carrier with peripheral seal – laboratory processed**
  A custom fabricated, laboratory processed carrier that covers the teeth and alveolar mucosa. Used as a vehicle to deliver prescribed medicaments for sustained contact with the gingiva, alveolar mucosa, and into the periodontal sulcus or pocket.

Revisions
One (1) procedure code

- ▲ **D5991** ~~topical~~ **vesiculobullous disease medicament carrier**
  A custom fabricated carrier that covers the teeth and alveolar mucosa, or alveolar mucosa alone, and is used to deliver ~~topical corticosteroids and similar effective~~ prescription medicaments for treatment ~~maximum sustained contact with the alveolar ridge and/or attached gingival tissues for the control and management~~ of immunologically mediated vesiculobullous ~~mucosal, chronic recurrent ulcerative, and other desquamative~~ diseases ~~of the gingiva and oral mucosa~~.

Deletions
None

D6000–D6199 VIII. Implant Services

Additions
Three (3) procedure codes

- **D6011 second stage implant surgery**
  Surgical access to an implant body for placement of a healing cap or to enable placement of an abutment.

- **D6013 surgical placement of mini implant**

- **D6052 semi-precision attachment abutment**
  Includes placement of keeper assembly.

Revisions
Two (2) procedure codes

▲ **D6010 surgical placement of implant body: endosteal implant**
  ~~Includes second stage surgery and placement of healing cap.~~

▲ **D6080 implant maintenance procedures when prostheses are removed and reinserted, including cleansing ~~removal~~ of prostheses ~~prosthesis, cleansing of prosthesis~~ and abutments ~~reinsertion of prosthesis~~**
  This procedure includes ~~a prophylaxis to provide~~ active debriding of the implant(s) and examination of all aspects of the implant system(s), including the occlusion and stability of the superstructure. The patient is also instructed in thorough daily cleansing of the implant(s). This is not a per implant code, and is indicated for implant supported fixed prostheses.

Deletions
None

D6200–D6999 IX. Prosthodontics, fixed

Additions
None

Revisions
None

Deletions
None

D7000-D7999   X. Oral and Maxillofacial Surgery

Additions
None

Revisions
Three (3) procedure codes

▲ **D7950   osseous, osteoperiosteal, or cartilage graft of the mandible or maxilla – autogenous or nonautogenous, by report**
This <u>procedure is</u> ~~code may be used~~ for ridge augmentation or reconstruction to increase height, width and/or volume of residual alveolar ridge. It includes obtaining ~~autograft, and/or allograft~~ <u>graft</u> material. Placement of a barrier membrane, if used, should be reported separately.

▲ **D7953   bone replacement graft for ridge preservation – per site**
~~Osseous autograft, allografts or non-osseous~~ <u>G</u>raft is placed in an extraction or implant removal site at the time of the extraction or removal to preserve ridge integrity (e.g., clinically indicated in preparation for implant reconstruction or where alveolar contour is critical to planned prosthetic reconstruction). <u>Does not include obtaining graft material.</u> Membrane, if used should be reported separately.

▲ **D7955   repair of maxillofacial soft and/or hard tissue defect**
Reconstruction of surgical, traumatic, or congenital defects of the facial bones, including the mandible, may utilize ~~autograft, allograft, or alloplastic~~ <u>graft</u> materials in conjunction with soft tissue procedures to repair and restore the facial bones to form and function. This does not include obtaining the graft and these procedures may require multiple surgical approaches. This procedure does not include edentulous maxilla and mandibular reconstruction for prosthetic considerations. ~~See code D7950.~~

Deletions
None

D8000-D8999 XI. Orthodontics

Additions
One (1) procedure code

- <u>D8694</u> <u>**repair of fixed retainers, includes reattachment**</u>

Revisions
One (1) procedure code

▲ **D8693 rebonding or recementing; ~~and/or repair, as required,~~ of fixed retainers**

Three (3) subcategories of service

▲ Limited Orthodontic Treatment

Orthodontic treatment with a limited objective, not <u>necessarily</u> involving the entire dentition. It may be directed at the only existing problem, or at only one aspect of a larger problem in which a decision is made to defer or forego more comprehensive therapy.

~~Examples of this type of treatment would be treatment in one arch only to correct crowding, partial treatment to open spaces or upright a tooth for a bridge or implant and partial treatment for closure of a space(s).~~

▲ Interceptive Orthodontic Treatment

~~Treatment using codes for interceptive orthodontic treatment are for procedures to lessen the severity or future effects of a malformation and to eliminate its cause.~~

<u>Interceptive orthodontics is an</u> ~~An~~ extension of preventive orthodontics that may include localized tooth movement. Such treatment may occur in the primary or transitional dentition and may include such procedures as the redirection of ectopically erupting teeth, correction of ~~isolated~~ dental crossbite or recovery of ~~recent minor~~ space loss where overall space is <u>ina</u>dequate. <u>When initiated during</u>   *(Continued)*

~~The key to successful interception is intervention in~~ the incipient stages of a developing problem, interceptive orthodontics may reduce ~~to lessen~~ the severity of the malformation and mitigate ~~eliminate~~ its cause. Complicating factors such as skeletal disharmonies, overall space deficiency, or other conditions may require subsequent ~~future~~ comprehensive therapy.

~~Early phases of comprehensive therapy may utilize some procedures that might also be used interceptively, but such procedures are not considered interceptive in those applications.~~

▲ Comprehensive Orthodontic Treatment

~~These codes should be used when there are multiple phases of treatment provided at different stages of dentofacial development.~~

~~For example, the use of an activator is generally stage one of a two-stage treatment. In this situation, placement of fixed appliances will generally be stage two of a two-stage treatment. Both phases should be listed as comprehensive treatment modified by the appropriate stage of dental development.~~

~~This is used to report the~~ Comprehensive orthodontic care includes a coordinated diagnosis and treatment leading to the improvement of a patient's craniofacial dysfunction and/or dentofacial deformity which may includ~~eing~~ anatomical, functional and/or a~~e~~sthetic relationships. Treatment ~~usually, but not necessarily,~~ may utilize~~s~~ fixed and/or removable orthodontic appliances and may also include functional and/or orthopedic appliances in growing and non-growing patients. Adjunctive procedures~~, such as extractions, maxillofacial surgery, nasopharyngeal surgery, myofunctional or speech therapy and restorative or periodontal care,~~ to facilitate care may be ~~coordinated disciplines~~ required. ~~Optimal care requires long-term consideration of patient's needs and periodic re-evaluation. Treatment~~ Comprehensive orthodontics may incorporate treatment ~~several~~ phases ~~with~~ focusing on specific objectives at various stages of ~~dental~~ dentofacial development.

Deletions
None

D9000-D9999 XII. Adjunctive General Services

Additions
One (1) procedure code

- **D9985** **sales tax**

Revisions
None

Deletions
None

3 Alphabetical Index to the CDT Code

ADA American Dental Association®

America's leading advocate for oral health

Alphabetic Index to the CDT Code

Term	Code(s)	Page(s)
A		
Abscess, incision and drainage, all types	D7510, D7511, D7520, D7521	72-73
Abutments	Also see **Retainers**	
for implants	D6051, D6056, D6057	56
Accession of tissue	D0472 – D0474	11
Acid etch; part of resin procedure	No separate code	
Adhesives, bonding agents (resin and amalgam bonding agents); part of restorative procedure	No separate code	
Adjunctive General Services (Category of Service)	D9000 – D9999	85-90
Adjunctive pre-diagnostic test	D0431	10
Adjust prosthetic appliance	D5992	52
Allograft, soft tissue	D4275, D7955	35, 79, 115
Alveoloplasty	D7310, D7311, D7320, D7321	70
Alveolus, fracture	D7670, D7671, D7770, D7771	74
Amalgam restorations	D2140 – D2161	17
Amalgam and resin bonding agents (part of restorative procedure)	No separate code	
Analgesia	D9230, D9241, D9242	86
non-intravenous conscious sedation	D9248	87
Anchorage device, temporary		
requiring flap	D7293	69
without flap	D7294	70
screw retained plate requiring flap	D7292	69

Alphabetical Index to the CDT Code

Term	Code(s)	Page(s)
Anesthesia		
general	D9220, D9221	85, 86
local	D9210, D9215	85
regional	D9211	85
trigeminal division block	D9212	85
Ankyloglossia	None	
Apexification/recalcification	D3351 – D3353	27-28, 102
Apexogenesis	D3222	26
Apically positioned flap	D4245	33
Apicoectomy	D3410 – D3426	28-29, 102
Appliance removal (not by dentist who placed)	D7997	80
Arthrocentesis	D7870	76
Arthroplasty	D7865	75
Arthroscopy	D7872 – D7877	76
Arthrotomy	D7860	75
Assessment of a patient	D0191	7
Athletic mouthguard	D9941	89
Autologous blood concentrate (collection and application)	D7921	77
B		
Bacteriologic studies	D0415	10
Behavior management	D9920	88
Biologic materials	D4265	34
in conjunction with periradicular surgery	D3431	29, 101

Term	Code(s)	Page(s)
Biopsy		
brush	D7288	69
hard tissue	D7285	69
soft tissue	D7286	69
Bitewing radiographs	D0270 – D0277	8
Bleaching		
external – per arch	D9972	90
external – per tooth	D9973	90
external bleaching for home application	D9975	90
internal – per tooth	D9974	90
Bone fragment (post-surgical removal)	D9930	89
Bone, harvest of	D7295	70
Bone tissue, excision	D7471 – D7490	72
Bonding agents; adhesives (resin and amalgam bonding agents)	No separate code – part of restorative procedure	
Bridge	See **Fixed Partial Dentures**	
Bruxism appliance	D9940	89

C

Term	Code(s)	Page(s)
Caries		
risk assessment	D0601 - D0603	13, 95
susceptibility test	D0425	10
Carrier		
fluoride gel	D5986	52

Alphabetical Index to the CDT Code

Term	Code(s)	Page(s)
periodontal medicament	D5994	53, 109
radiation	D5983	52
vesiculobolus medicament	D5991	53, 109
Case presentation	D9450	87
Cast post and core	D2952	22
each additional (same tooth)	D2953	22
Casts, diagnostic (study models)	D0470	11
Cephalometric image	D0340	8
Collection and application of autologous blood concentrate	D7921	77
Combined connective tissue and double pedicle graft	D4276	35
Complications, post-surgical	D9930	89
Composite resin	**See Resin-based composite** (direct and indirect)	
Comprehensive orthodontics	D8070 – D8090	82
Condylectomy	D7840	75
Cone Beam – CT		
image capture and interpretation	D0364 – D0368	8-9
image capture only	D0380 – D0384	9
interpretation and report only	D0391	9
post processing image or image sets	D0393 – D0395	10
Connector bar		
dental implant supported	D6055	56
fixed partial denture	D6920	66

 © 2013 American Dental Association

Term	Code(s)	Page(s)
Conscious sedation	D9241, D9242, D9248	86-87
Consultation	D9310	87
Coping	D2975, D6975	23, 66
Core buildup	D2950	22
Coronectomy	D7251	68
Coronoidectomy	D7991	80
Counseling		
nutritional	D1310	15
tobacco	D1320	15
oral hygiene	D1330	15
Crevicular antimicrobial agents	D4381	37
Crown		
abutment (on implant) supported	D6058 – D6064, D6094	57-58
implant supported	D6065 – D6067	58-59
individual restorations (indirect)	D2710 – D2799	20
prefabricated	D2929 – D2934	21
provisional	D2799	20
recement	D2920	21
repair	D2980	23
resin-based composite, anterior, direct	D2390	18
temporary (fractured tooth)	D2970	22
under existing removable partial	D2971	23

Alphabetical Index to the CDT Code

Term	Code(s)	Page(s)
Crown exposure	D4230, D4231	32
Crown lengthening, hard tissue	D4249	33
Crown repair	D2980	23
Cryosurgery	D7465	71
Culture and sensitivity test	D0415	10
Culture, viral	D0416	10
Curettage		
open flap	D4240, D4241	32
without flap	D4341, D4342	36
Cysts, removal of	D7410 – D7465	71
Cytologic smears	D0480	11
Cytology sample collection	D7287	69

D

Debridement		
endodontic	D3221	25
full mouth	D4355	37
periimplant	D6101 – D6102	56
Dentures (removable)		
adjustments	D5410 – D5422	40
complete	D5110 – D5120	39
immediate, complete	D5130, D5140	39
implant/abutment supported, complete	D6053	57
implant/abutment supported, partial	D6054	57

Term	Code(s)	Page(s)
modification of removable prosthesis following implant surgery	D5875	42
overdenture	D5863 – D5866	42, 107
partial	D5211 – D5281	39–40
precision attachment	D5862	42
rebase	D5710 – D5721	41
reline	D5730 – D5761	41
repairs, complete and partial	D5510, D5520, D5610 – D5671	40
temporary/interim	D5810 – D5821	41–42
Dentures (fixed)		
implant/abutment supported, full	D6078	57
implant/abutment supported, partial	D6079	57
Desensitizing medicament	D9910	88
Desensitizing resin	D9911	88
Destruction of lesion	D7465	71
Diagnostic (Category of Service)	D0100 – D0999	5–13
Diagnostic casts	D0470	11
Diagnostic imaging		
image capture and interpretation	D0210 – D0371	7–9
image capture only	D0380 – D0386	9
interpretation and report only	D0391	9
post processing image or image sets	D0393 – D0395	10, 95
Disc repair (TMJ)	D7852	75
Dietary planning (nutritional counseling)	D1310	15

Term	Code(s)	Page(s)
Distal/proximal wedge	D4274	35
Dressing change, periodontal, unscheduled	D4920	37, 105
Drugs		
therapeutic parenteral, single administration	D9610	88
therapeutic parental, two or more administrations	D9612	88
other	D9630	88
Dry socket/localized osteitis	D9930	89

E

Emergency treatment	D0140, D9110	5, 85
Enamel microabrasion	D9970	89
Enameloplasty	D9971	90
Endodontics (Category of Service)	D3000 – D3999	25-30
Endodontic endosseous implant	D3460	29
Equilibration (occlusal adjustment)	D9951, D9952	89
Eruption of teeth		
mobilization, surgical	D7282	68
placement of device to aid eruption	D7283	69
Evaluations		
periodic – established patient	D0120	5
limited – problem focused	D0140	5
for patient under 3 years & counseling with primary caregiver	D0145	5

Term	Code(s)	Page(s)
comprehensive – new or established patient	D0150	6
detailed and extensive – problem focused, by report	D0160	6
re-evaluation – limited	D0170	6
comprehensive periodontal – new or established patient	D0180	7
Excision		
benign lesion	D7410 – D7412	71
malignant lesion/tumor	D7413 – D7415, D7440, D7441	71
Exfoliative cytological smear	D0480	11
Exostosis (tuberosity); removal of		
lateral exostosis	D7471	72
osseous tuberosity	D7485	72
surgical reduction of fibrous tuberosity	D7972	79
torus palatinus	D7472	72
torus mandibularis	D7473	72
Extraoral Images (radiographic)	D0250, D0260	8
Extractions	D7111, D7140	67
surgical	D7210 – D7250	67-68

F

Facial Bone Survey	D0290	8
Fiberotomy, transseptal	D7291	69
Fibroma	D7410, D7411	71
Fissurotomy	see **Odontoplasty**	

Alphabetical Index to the CDT Code

Term	Code(s)	Page(s)
Fistula		
oroantral	D7260	68
salivary	D7983	79
Fixation device, not in conjunction with fracture	D7998	80
Fixed partial dentures (bridges)		
pontics	D6205 – D6253	63
recementation	D6930	66
repair	D6980	66
retainers		
crowns	D6710 – D6794	65
implant/abutment supported	D6068 – D6077, D6194	59-60
inlay/onlay	D6600 – D6634	64
Maryland Bridge	D6545, D6548	64
pediatric	D6985	66
sectioning	D9120	85
Flaps		
apically positioned	D4245	33
gingival	D4240, D4241	32
Flexible base partial denture	D5225, D5226	39-40
"Flipper", interim/transitional removable prosthesis (aka "stayplate")	D5820, D5821	42
Fluoride		
dispensing for home use	D9630	88

Term	Code(s)	Page(s)
gel carrier	D5986	52
topical	D1208	15
varnish	D1206	15
Foreign bodies, removal of	D7530, D7540	73
Fractures, treatment of		
Alveolus	D7670, D7770	74
facial bone	D7680, D7780	74
malar/zygomatic arch,		
no incision required	D7650 – D7660	73
surgical incision required	D7750 – D7760	74
mandible		
compound open reduction	D7730	74
compound closed reduction	D7740	74
simple open reduction	D7630	73
simple closed reduction	D7640	73
maxilla		
compound open reduction	D7710	74
compound closed reduction	D7720	74
simple open reduction	D7610	73
simple closed reduction	D7620	73
Frenectomy/frenotomy (frenulectomy)	D7960	79
Frenuloplasty	D7963	79
Full mouth series	D0210	7

Term	Code(s)	Page(s)
G		
Genetic test	D0421	10
Gingiva, pericoronal, removal of	D7971	79
Gingival flap	D4240, D4241	32
Gingival Irrigation	D4921	37, 105
Gingivectomy/gingivoplasty	D4210, D4211, D4212	31-32
Glass ionomers (resin restorations)	D2330 – D2394	18
Gold foil	D2410 – D2430	18
Graft		
bone replacement	D4263, D4264, D6103, D6104, D7953	33-34, 56, 78, 105, 115
combined connective tissue and double pedicle	D4276	35
free soft tissue	D4277 – D4278	35-36
maxillofacial soft/hard tissue	D7955	78, 115
osseous, osteoperiosteal, or cartilage	D7950	78
pedicle soft tissue	D4270	35
periradicular	D3428, D3429	29, 101
sinus augmentation	D7951	78
skin	D7920	77
soft tissue	D4270 – D4273	35
subepithelial connective tissue	D4273	35
synthetic	D7955	79, 115
Guided tissue regeneration	D4266, D4267	34
in conjunction with periradicular surgery	D3432	29, 101

Term	Code(s)	Page(s)
H		
Harvest of bone	D7295	70
Hemisection	D3920	30
Hospital call (hospital or ambulatory surgicenter visit)	D9420	87
House call (nursing home visit)	D9410	87
Hyperplastic tissue removal	D7970	79
I		
Images, oral/facial	D0350	8, 96
Immediate complete denture	D5130, D5140	39
Impacted tooth, removal of	D7220 – D7241	67-68
Implant		
abutments	D6056, D6057, D6051	56
chin	D7995	80
endodontic	D3460	29
endosteal/endosseous	D6010	55, 111
eposteal/subperiosteal	D6040	55
interim implant	D6012	55
maintenance	D6080	61, 111
mandible	D7996	80
mini	D6013	55, 111
modification of removable prosthesis	D5875	42
other implant services	D6080 – D6199	61, 111

Alphabetical Index to the CDT Code

Term	Code(s)	Page(s)
peri-implant defect	D6103	56
radiographic/surgical implant index	D6190	55
recement	D6092, D6093	61
removal	D6100	56
repair	D6090, D6091, D6095	61
second stage surgery	D6011	55, 111
transosteal/transosseous	D6050	56
Implant Services (Category of Service)	D6000 – D6199	55-61
Implantation (of tooth)	See **Reimplantation**	
Incision and drainage	D7510, D7511, D7520, D7521	72-73
Inlay		
fixed partial denture retainers		
metallic	D6602 – D6607, D6624	64
porcelain/ceramic	D6600 – D6601	64
metallic	D2510 – D2530	19
porcelain/ceramic	D2610 – D2630	19
recement inlay	D2910	21
resin-based composite	D2650 – D2652	19
Intentional reimplantation	D3470	29
Interceptive orthodontics	D8050, D8060	82
Interim abutment	D6051	56
Interim complete denture	D5810, D5811	41
Interim partial denture	D5820, D5821	42

Term	Code(s)	Page(s)
Internal root repair	D3333	27
Interpretation of diagnostic image (different practitioner)	D0391	9
Intravenous conscious sedation/analgesia		
first 30 minutes	D9241	86
each additional 15 minutes	D9242	86
Irrigation (gingival)	D4921	37, 105

J

Joint reconstruction	D7858	75

K

No "K" terms		

L

Labial veneer	D2960, D2961, D2962	22
Laser	No separate code – part of dental procedure code that appropriately describes the service provided	
Lateral exostosis	D7471	72
LeFort I, osteotomy	D7946, D7947	77-78
II, osteotomy	D7948, D7949	78
III, osteotomy	D7948, D7949	78
Lesions, surgical excision		
intra-osseous lesions	D7440 – D7461	70-71
soft tissue	D7410 – D7415, D7465	71
Limited orthodontic treatment	D8010 – D8040	81

Alphabetical Index to the CDT Code

Term	Code(s)	Page(s)
Localized osteitis/dry socket	D9930	89

M

Term	Code(s)	Page(s)
Maintenance and cleaning of prosthesis	D5993	52
Malar bone, repair of fracture	D7650, D7660, D7750, D7760	73-74
Malocclusion, correction of	D8000 – D8999	81-83
Mandible, fracture of	D7630 – D7640, D7730 – D7740	73-74
Maryland Bridge (resin bonded fixed prosthesis)		
retainer/abutment	D6545, D6548	64
pontic	D6210 – D6252	63
Maxilla, repair of fracture	D7610 – D7620, D7710 – D7720	73-74
Maxillofacial defect	D7955	79, 115
Maxillofacial MRI		
capture and interpretation	D0369	9
image capture (only)	D0385	9
Maxillofacial Prosthetics (Category of Service)	D5900 - D5999	43-53
adjust prosthetic appliance	D5992	52
maintenance and cleaning of prosthesis	D5993	52
Maxillofacial ultrasound		
capture and interpretation	D0370	9
image capture (only)	D0386	9
Metals, classification of		4
Microabrasion, enamel	D9970	89

Term	Code(s)	Page(s)
Microorganisms, culture and sensitivity	D0415	10
Moulage, facial	D5911, D5912	43
Mouthguard, athletic	D9941	89
Mucosal abnormalities, pre-diagnostic test	D0431	10
Myotomy	D7856	75
N		
Neoplasms, removal of	D7410 – D7465	71
Nightguard	D9940	89
Nitrous oxide, analgesia	D9230	86
Non-intravenous conscious sedation	D9248	87
Non-odontogenic cyst	D7460, D7461	72
Nursing home, (house/extended care facility visit)	D9410	87
Nutritional counseling	D1310	15
O		
Obturator		
post surgical	D5932	46
refitting	D5933	47
surgical	D5931	46
Occlusal adjustment (equilibration)	D9951, D9952	89
Occlusal image, intraoral	D0240	7
Occlusal guard	D9940	89
reline or repair	D9942	89

Alphabetical Index to the CDT Code

Term	Code(s)	Page(s)
Occlusal orthotic device	D7880	76
Occlusion analysis	D9950	89
Odontogenic cyst	D7450, D7451	72
Odontoplasty (enameloplasty)	D9971	90
Office visit	D9430, D9440	87
Onlay		
fixed partial denture retainers, metallic	D6610 – D6615, D6634	64
metallic	D2542 – D2544	19
porcelain/ceramic	D2642 – D2644	19
resin-based composite	D2662 – D2664	19
Operculectomy	D7971	79
Oral & Maxillofacial Surgery (Category of Service)	D7000 – D7999	67-80
Oral hygiene instructions	D1330	15
Oral pathology		
accession of tissue	D0472 – D0474; D0480, D0486	11
consultation, slides	D0484, D0485	12
cytology	D0480	11
decalcification procedure	D0475	11
electron microscopy	D0481	12
immunofluorescence		
direct	D0482	12
indirect	D0483	12
immunohistochemical stains	D0478	12

 © 2013 American Dental Association

Term	Code(s)	Page(s)
other oral pathology procedures	D0502	13
special stains	D0476, D0477	12
tissue hybridization	D0479	12
Orthodontics (Category of Service)	D8000 – D8999	81-83
Orthodontic treatment (not by the original treating dentist)	D8690	83
Orthotic appliance	D7880	76
Osseous surgery/graft	D4260 – D4264	33-34, 105
Ostectomy, partial	D7550	73
Osteitis, localized; dry socket	D9930	89
Osteoplasty	D7940	77
Osteotomy	D7941 – D7945	77
Overdenture		
maxillary	D5863, D5864	42, 107
mandibular	D5865, D5866	42, 107
dental implant supported fixed	D6078, D6079	57
dental implant supported removable	D6053, D6054	57

P

Palliative treatment	D9110	85
Panoramic image	D0330	8
Partial dentures, fixed	See **fixed partial denture**	
Partial dentures, removable		
adjustments	D5421, D5422	40

Alphabetical Index to the CDT Code

Term	Code(s)	Page(s)
cast metal framework, resin base	D5213, D5214	39
flexible base	D5225, D5226	39-40
implant/abutment supported	D6054	57
interim	D5820, D5821	42
overdenture	D5863-D5866	42, 107
reline	D5740, D5741, D5760, D5761	41
repair	D5610 – D5671	40
resin base	D5211, D5212	39
unilateral	D5281	40
Patient		
Screening	D0190	7
Assessment	D0191	7
Perforation defect, internal repair	D3333	27
Periapical images	D0220 - D0230	7
Pericoronal gingival excision	D7971	79
Periodic orthodontic visit	D8670	83
Periodontal evaluation	D0180	7
Periodontal maintenance	D4910	37
Periodontics (Category of Service)	D4000 – D4999	31-37
Periradicular surgery/apicoectomy	D3410 – D3426	28-29, 102
Periradicular surgery without apicoectomy	D3427	29, 101
Pharmacologic agents	See **Drugs**	
Photographic images, diagnostic	D0350	8, 96

Term	Code(s)	Page(s)
Pin retention	D2951	22
Pit and fissure sealant	D1351	16
Plasma rich protein	D4265	34
Porcelain/ceramic, definition of		4
Post and core		
indirectly fabricated	D2952	22
each additional (same tooth)	D2953	22
prefabricated	D2954	22
each additional (same tooth)	D2957	22
Post, removal of	D2955	22
Precision attachment	D5862, D6950	42, 66
Replacement of replaceable part	D5867, D6091	42, 61
Prefabricated crown	D2929 – D2933	21
Pre-orthodontic treatment visit	D8660	83
Preventive (Category of Service)	D1000 – D1999	15-16, 97
Preventive resin restoration	D1352	16
Prophylaxis	D1110, D1120	15
Prostheses (maxillofacial prosthetics)	D5900 – D5999	43-53
auricular	D5914	43
cranial	D5924	45
facial	D5919, D5925, D5929	44-46
feeding aid	D5951	48
maintenance and cleaning	D5993	52

Alphabetical Index to the CDT Code

Term	Code(s)	Page(s)
mandibular resection	D5934, D5935	47
nasal	D5913, D5922, D5926	43, 44
oburator	D5931 – D5933, D5936	46, 47
ocular	D5916	44
orbital	D5915	44
palatal	D5954 – D5959	49-50
speech aid	D5952, D5953, D5960	49-50
Prosthodontics		
fixed (Category of Service)	D6200 – D6999	63-66
implant-supported	D6053 – D6079, D6094, D6194	57-58, 60
maxillofacial (Category of Service)	D5900 – D5999	43-53
removable (Category of Service)	D5000 – D5899	39-42
Protective restoration	D2940	21
Provisional		
single crown	D2799	20
pontic (FPD)	D6253	63
retainer crown (FPD)	D6793	65
Proximal/distal wedge	D4274	35
Pulp cap	D3110, D3120	25
Pulp vitality tests	D0460	10
Pulpal debridement	D3221	25
Pupal regeneration	D3355 – D3357	28, 102
Pulpal therapy, primary teeth	D3230, D3240	26

Term	Code(s)	Page(s)
Pulpotomy		
therapeutic (excluding final restoration)	D3220	25
partial for apexogenesis	D3222	26
Q		
No "Q" terms.		
R		
Radiation		
carrier	D5983	52
cone locator	D5985	51
shield	D5984	51
Radiographic/surgical implant index	D6190	55
Radiographs		
image capture and interpretation	D0210 – D0340	7-8
interpretation and report only	D0391	9
Reattach tooth fragment	D2921	21, 99
Recalcification/apexification	D3351 – D3353	27-28
Recement		
bridge	D6930	66
crown	D2920	21
fixed retainers	D8693	83, 117
implant fixed partial denture	D6093	61
implant crown	D6092	61
inlay	D2910	21

Alphabetical Index to the CDT Code

Term	Code(s)	Page(s)
onlay	D2910	21
post and core	D2915	21
space maintainer	D1550	16
veneer	D2910	21
Reimplantation		
intentional	D3470	29
accidentally evulsed or displaced	D7270	68
Removable partial denture	See **Partial Dentures**	
Repair		
complete removable denture	D5510, D5520	40
crown	D2980	23
fixed partial denture	D6980	66
implant precision or semi-precision attachment	D6091	61
inlay	D2981	23
occlusal guard	D9942	89
onlay	D2982	23
orthodontic appliance	D8691	83
orthodontic fixed retainer	D8693, D8694	83, 117
precision or semi-precision attachment	D5867, D6052	42, 57, 112
removable partial dentures	D5610 - D5671	40
veneer	D2983	23
Resin, definition of		4

Term	Code(s)	Page(s)
Resin-based composite, direct		
anterior	D2330 – D2335	18
crown	D2390	18
posterior	D2391 – D2394	18
veneers	D2960	22
Resin-based composite, indirect		
crown	D2710	20
fixed partial denture abutment	D6710	65
inlay/onlay	D2650 – D2664	19
pontic	D6205	63
¾ crown	D2712	20
veneers	D2961	22
Restorations		
amalgam	D2140 – D2161	17
gold foil	D2410 – D2430	18
inlay/onlay	D2510 – D2664,	19
	D6600 – D6634	64
interim therapeutic	D2941	21, 99
resin-based composite	D2330 – D2394	18
resin infiltration	D2990	21
preventive resin	D1352	16
protective	D2940	21
Restorative (Category of Service)	D2000 – D2999	17-23

Alphabetical Index to the CDT Code

Term	Code(s)	Page(s)
Restorative foundation for indirect restoration	D2949	22, 99
Retainers		
fixed partial denture		
resin bonded (aka "Maryland Bridge")	D6545, D6548	64
inlays/onlays	D6600 – D6634	64
crowns	D6710 – D6794	65
implant abutment supported	D6068 – D6074, D6194	59-60
implant supported	D6075 – D6077	60
orthodontic	D8680, D8691, D8692	83
Retreatment, endodontic	D3346 – D3348	27
Retrograde filling	D3430	29
Revision, periodontal surgery	D4268	34
Ridge augmentation (grafting)	D7950	78, 115
Root		
planing	D4341	36
removal	D7140, D7250	67-68
resection/amputation	D3450	29
Root canal		
therapy	D3310 – D3353	26-28
obstruction	D3331	27
incomplete	D3332	27
Rubber dam, surgical isolation	D3910	30

Term	Code(s)	Page(s)
S		
Sales tax	D9985	90, 119
Saliva		
sample collection	D0417	10
analysis of sample	D0418	10
Salivary gland		
excision	D7981	79
fistula closure	D7983	79
Scaling and root planing	D4341, D4342	36
Screening of a patient	D0190	7
Sealant	D1351	16
Section of fixed partial denture	D9120	85
Sedation		
deep	D9220, D9221	85–86
intravenous, conscious	D9241, D9242	86
non-intravenous, conscious	D9248	87
Sedative filling	See **Protective Restoration**	
Semi-precision attachment abutment	D6052	57, 111
Sequestrectomy	D7550	73
Sialodochoplasty	D7982	79
Sialoendoscopy capture and interpretation	D0371	9
Sialography	D0310	8

Alphabetical Index to the CDT Code

Term	Code(s)	Page(s)
onlay, FPD retainer	D6634	64
pontic	D6214	63
Tobacco counseling	D1320	15
Tomographic survey	D0322	8
Tongue thrusting appliance	D8210, D8220	83
Tooth, natural		
caries susceptibility test	D0425	10
extraction	D7111, D7140, D7210 – D7250	67-68
impacted, removal of	D7220 – D7241	67-68
intentional reimplantation	D3470	29
pulp vitality test	D0460	10
reimplantation, evulsed/displaced	D7270	68
surgical access	D7280	68
surgical repositioning	D7290	69
transplantation	D7272	68
Tooth, reattach fragment	D2921	21, 99
Topical medicament carrier	D5991	53, 109
Torus (removal of)		
mandibularis	D7473	72
palatinus	D7472	72
Tracheotomy, emergency	D7990	80
Transplantation, tooth	D7272	68

Term	Code(s)	Page(s)
Transseptal fiberotomy	D7291	69
Trismus appliance	D5937	48
Tuberosity		
fibrous	D7972	79
surgical reduction	D7485	72
Tumors, (removal of)	D7440 – D7465	71
U		
Unerupted tooth, surgical access	D7280	68
Unilateral removable partial denture	D5281	40
V		
Veneers	D2960 – D2962	22
Vertical bitewings	D0277	8
Vestibuloplasty	D7340, D7350	71
Viral culture	D0416	10
W		
Wax-up (diagnostic)	D9950	89
Whitening	See **Bleaching**	
Wounds, treatment of	D7910 – D7912	76-77
X		
X-rays	See **Diagnostic Imaging**	

Alphabetical Index to the CDT Code

Term	Code(s)	Page(s)
Y		
No "Y" terms.		
Z		
Zygomatic arch		
simple fracture treatment		
open reduction	D7650	73
closed reduction	D7660	74
compound fracture treatment		
open reduction	D7750	74
closed reduction	D7760	74

4 Numeric Index to the CDT Code

ADA American Dental Association®

America's leading advocate for oral health

CDT Code	Page in CDT Manual Section		Change Legend – ● = Addition ▲ = Revision
	1 – Current Version	2 – Change Summary	

I. Diagnostic

CDT Code	1 – Current Version	2 – Change Summary	Change Legend
D0120	5		
D0140	5		
D0145	5		
D0150	6		
D0160	6		
D0170	6		
D0180	7		
D0190	7		
D0191	7		
D0210	7		
D0220	7		
D0230	7		
D0240	8		
D0250	8		
D0260	8		
D0270	8		
D0272	8		
D0273	8		
D0274	8		
D0277	8		
D0290	8		
D0310	8		
D0320	8		
D0321	8		
D0322	8		
D0330	8		
D0340	8		
D0350	8	96	▲
D0364	8		
D0365	8		
D0366	8		

© 2013 American Dental Association

CDT Code	Page in CDT Manual Section		Change Legend – • = Addition ▲ = Revision
	1 – Current Version	2 – Change Summary	
D0367	9		
D0368	9		
D0369	9		
D0370	9		
D0371	9		
D0380	9		
D0381	9		
D0382	9		
D0383	9		
D0384	9		
D0385	9		
D0386	9		
D0391	9		
D0393	10	95	•
D0394	10	95	•
D0395	10	95	•
D0415	10		
D0416	10		
D0417	10		
D0418	10		
D0421	10		
D0425	10		
D0431	10		
D0460	10		
D0470	11		
D0472	11		
D0473	11		
D0474	11		
D0475	11		
D0476	12		
D0477	12		
D0478	12		
D0479	12		
D0480	11		

| CDT Code | Page in CDT Manual Section | | Change Legend – ● = Addition ▲ = Revision |
	1 - Current Version	2 - Change Summary	
D0481	12		
D0482	12		
D0483	12		
D0484	12		
D0485	12		
D0486	11		
D0502	13		
D0601	13	95	●
D0602	13	95	●
D0603	13	95	●
D0999	13		

II. Preventive

D1110	15		
D1120	15		
D1206	15		
D1208	15		
D1310	15		
D1320	15		
D1330	15		
D1351	16		
D1352	16		
D1510	16		
D1515	16		
D1520	16		
D1525	16		
D1550	16		
D1555	16		
D1999	16	97	●

III. Restorative

D2140	17		
D2150	17		
D2160	17		

© 2013 American Dental Association

CDT Code	Page in CDT Manual Section		Change Legend – • = Addition ▲ = Revision
	1 - Current Version	2 - Change Summary	
D2161	17		
D2330	18		
D2331	18		
D2332	18		
D2335	18		
D2390	18		
D2391	18		
D2392	18		
D2393	18		
D2394	18		
D2410	18		
D2420	18		
D2430	18		
D2510	19		
D2520	19		
D2530	19		
D2542	19		
D2543	19		
D2544	19		
D2610	19		
D2620	19		
D2630	19		
D2642	19		
D2643	19		
D2644	19		
D2650	19		
D2651	19		
D2652	19		
D2662	19		
D2663	19		
D2664	19		
D2710	20		
D2712	20		
D2720	20		

CDT Code	Page in CDT Manual Section		Change Legend – • = Addition ▲ = Revision
	1 – Current Version	2 – Change Summary	
D2721	20		
D2722	20		
D2740	20		
D2750	20		
D2751	20		
D2752	20		
D2780	20		
D2781	20		
D2782	20		
D2783	20		
D2790	20		
D2791	20		
D2792	20		
D2794	20		
D2799	20		
D2910	21		
D2915	21		
D2920	21		
D2921	21	99	•
D2929	21		
D2930	21		
D2931	21		
D2932	21		
D2933	21		
D2934	21		
D2940	21		
D2941	21	99	•
D2949	22	99	•
D2950	22	99	▲
D2951	22		
D2952	22		
D2953	22		
D2954	22		
D2955	22		

© 2013 American Dental Association

| CDT Code | Page in CDT Manual Section | | Change Legend – • = Addition ▲ = Revision |
	1 - Current Version	2 - Change Summary	
D2957	22		
D2960	22		
D2961	22		
D2962	22		
D2970	22		
D2971	23		
D2975	23		
D2980	23		
D2981	23		
D2982	23		
D2983	23		
D2990	21		
D2999	23		

IV. Endodontics

CDT Code	1 - Current Version	2 - Change Summary	Change Legend
D3110	25		
D3120	25		
D3220	25		
D3221	25		
D3222	26		
D3230	26		
D3240	26		
D3310	26		
D3320	26		
D3330	26		
D3331	27		
D3332	27		
D3333	27		
D3346	27		
D3347	27		
D3348	27		
D3351	27	102	▲
D3352	27	102	▲
D3353	28		

| CDT Code | Page in CDT Manual Section | | Change Legend – • = Addition ▲ = Revision |
	1 – Current Version	2 – Change Summary	
D3355	28	101	•
D3356	28	101	•
D3357	28	101	•
D3410	28	102	▲
D3421	28	102	▲
D3425	28	102	▲
D3426	29	102	▲
D3427	29	101	•
D3428	29	101	•
D3429	29	101	•
D3430	29		
D3431	29	101	•
D3432	29	101	•
D3450	29		
D3460	29		
D3470	29		
D3910	30		
D3920	30		
D3950	30		
D3999	30		

V. Periodontics

CDT Code	1 – Current Version	2 – Change Summary	Change Legend
D4210	31		
D4211	31		
D4212	32		
D4230	32		
D4231	32		
D4240	32		
D4241	32		
D4245	33		
D4249	33		
D4260	33		
D4261	33		
D4263	33	105	▲

CDT Code	Page in CDT Manual Section		Change Legend – ● = Addition ▲ = Revision
	1 – Current Version	2 – Change Summary	
D4264	34	105	▲
D4265	34		
D4266	34		
D4267	34		
D4268	34		
D4270	35		
D4273	35		
D4274	35		
D4275	35		
D4276	35		
D4277	35		
D4278	36		
D4320	36		
D4321	36		
D4341	36		
D4342	36		
D4355	37		
D4381	37		
D4910	37		
D4920	37	105	▲
D4921	37	105	●
D4999	37		

VI. Prosthodontics (removable)

CDT Code	Page in CDT Manual Section		
D5110	39		
D5120	39		
D5130	39		
D5140	39		
D5211	39		
D5212	39		
D5213	39		
D5214	39		
D5225	39		
D5226	40		

© 2013 American Dental Association

| CDT Code | Page in CDT Manual Section | | Change Legend – • = Addition ▲ = Revision |
	1 – Current Version	2 – Change Summary	
D5281	40		
D5410	40		
D5411	40		
D5421	40		
D5422	40		
D5510	40		
D5520	40		
D5610	40		
D5620	40		
D5630	40		
D5640	40		
D5650	40		
D5660	40		
D5670	40		
D5671	40		
D5710	41		
D5711	41		
D5720	41		
D5721	41		
D5730	41		
D5731	41		
D5740	41		
D5741	41		
D5750	41		
D5751	41		
D5760	41		
D5761	41		
D5810	41		
D5811	41		
D5820	42		
D5821	42		
D5850	42		
D5851	42		
D5862	42		

| CDT Code | Page in CDT Manual Section | | Change Legend – • = Addition ▲ = Revision |
	1 - Current Version	2 - Change Summary	
D5863	42	107	•
D5864	42	107	•
D5865	42	107	•
D5866	42	107	•
D5867	42		
D5875	42		
D5899	42		

VII. Maxillofacial Prosthetics

D5911	43		
D5912	43		
D5913	43		
D5914	43		
D5915	44		
D5916	44		
D5919	44		
D5922	44		
D5923	45		
D5924	45		
D5925	45		
D5926	45		
D5927	45		
D5928	46		
D5929	46		
D5931	46		
D5932	46		
D5933	47		
D5934	47		
D5935	47		
D5936	48		
D5937	48		
D5951	48		
D5952	49		
D5953	49		

| CDT Code | Page in CDT Manual Section | | Change Legend –
 ● = Addition
 ▲ = Revision |
	1 – Current Version	2 – Change Summary	
D5954	49		
D5955	50		
D5958	50		
D5959	50		
D5960	50		
D5982	51		
D5983	52		
D5984	51		
D5985	51		
D5986	52		
D5987	51		
D5988	52		
D5991	53	109	▲
D5992	52		
D5993	52		
D5994	53	109	●
D5999	53		

VIII. Implant Services

CDT Code	1 – Current Version	2 – Change Summary	
D6010	55	111	▲
D6011	55	111	●
D6012	55		
D6013	55	111	●
D6040	55		
D6050	56		
D6051	56		
D6052	57	111	●
D6053	57		
D6054	57		
D6055	56		
D6056	56		
D6057	56		
D6058	57		
D6059	57		

| CDT Code | Page in CDT Manual Section | | Change Legend – ● = Addition ▲ = Revision |
	1 - Current Version	2 - Change Summary	
D6060	58		
D6061	58		
D6062	58		
D6063	58		
D6064	58		
D6065	58		
D6066	59		
D6067	59		
D6068	59		
D6069	59		
D6070	59		
D6071	59		
D6072	59		
D6073	60		
D6074	60		
D6075	60		
D6076	60		
D6077	60		
D6078	57		
D6079	57		
D6080	61	111	▲
D6090	61		
D6091	61		
D6092	61		
D6093	61		
D6094	58		
D6095	61		
D6100	56		
D6101	56		
D6102	56		
D6103	56		
D6104	56		
D6190	55		
D6194	60		

 © 2013 American Dental Association

| CDT Code | Page in CDT Manual Section | | Change Legend – • = Addition ▲ = Revision |
	1 – Current Version	2 – Change Summary	
D6199	61		

IX. Prosthodontics, Fixed

D6205	63		
D6210	63		
D6211	63		
D6212	63		
D6214	63		
D6240	63		
D6241	63		
D6242	63		
D6245	63		
D6250	63		
D6251	63		
D6252	63		
D6253	63		
D6545	64		
D6548	64		
D6600	64		
D6601	64		
D6602	64		
D6603	64		
D6604	64		
D6605	64		
D6606	64		
D6607	64		
D6608	64		
D6609	64		
D6610	64		
D6611	64		
D6612	64		
D6613	64		
D6614	64		
D6615	64		

| CDT Code | Page in CDT Manual Section | | Change Legend – • = Addition ▲ = Revision |
	1 - Current Version	2 - Change Summary	
D6624	64		
D6634	64		
D6710	65		
D6720	65		
D6721	65		
D6722	65		
D6740	65		
D6750	65		
D6751	65		
D6752	65		
D6780	65		
D6781	65		
D6782	65		
D6783	65		
D6790	65		
D6791	65		
D6792	65		
D6793	65		
D6794	65		
D6920	66		
D6930	66		
D6940	66		
D6950	66		
D6975	66		
D6980	66		
D6985	66		
D6999	66		

X. Oral and Maxillofacial Surgery

CDT Code	Page in CDT Manual Section		
D7111	67		
D7140	67		
D7210	67		
D7220	67		
D7230	67		

CDT Code	Page in CDT Manual Section		Change Legend – • = Addition ▲ = Revision
	1 – Current Version	2 – Change Summary	
D7240	67		
D7241	68		
D7250	68		
D7251	68		
D7260	68		
D7261	68		
D7270	68		
D7272	68		
D7280	68		
D7282	68		
D7283	69		
D7285	69		
D7286	69		
D7287	69		
D7288	69		
D7290	69		
D7291	69		
D7292	69		
D7293	69		
D7294	70		
D7295	70		
D7310	70		
D7311	70		
D7320	70		
D7321	70		
D7340	71		
D7350	71		
D7410	71		
D7411	71		
D7412	71		
D7413	71		
D7414	71		
D7415	71		
D7440	71		

© 2013 American Dental Association

CDT Code	Page in CDT Manual Section		Change Legend – • = Addition ▲ = Revision
	1 – Current Version	2 – Change Summary	
D7441	71		
D7450	72		
D7451	72		
D7460	72		
D7461	72		
D7465	71		
D7471	72		
D7472	72		
D7473	72		
D7485	72		
D7490	72		
D7510	72		
D7511	72		
D7520	72		
D7521	73		
D7530	73		
D7540	73		
D7550	73		
D7560	73		
D7610	73		
D7620	73		
D7630	73		
D7640	73		
D7650	73		
D7660	73		
D7670	74		
D7671	74		
D7680	74		
D7710	74		
D7720	74		
D7730	74		
D7740	74		
D7750	74		
D7760	74		

 © 2013 American Dental Association

CDT Code	Page in CDT Manual Section		Change Legend – • = Addition ▲ = Revision
	1 - Current Version	2 - Change Summary	
D7770	74		
D7771	74		
D7780	74		
D7810	75		
D7820	75		
D7830	75		
D7840	75		
D7850	75		
D7852	75		
D7854	75		
D7856	75		
D7858	75		
D7860	75		
D7865	75		
D7870	76		
D7871	76		
D7872	76		
D7873	76		
D7874	76		
D7875	76		
D7876	76		
D7877	76		
D7880	76		
D7899	76		
D7910	76		
D7911	77		
D7912	77		
D7920	77		
D7921	77		
D7940	77		
D7943	77		
D7944	77		
D7945	77		
D7946	77		

CDT Code	Page in CDT Manual Section		Change Legend – • = Addition ▲ = Revision
	1 – Current Version	2 – Change Summary	
D7947	78		
D7948	78		
D7949	78		
D7950	78	115	▲
D7951	78		
D7952	78		
D7953	78	115	▲
D7955	79	115	▲
D7960	79		
D7963	79		
D7970	79		
D7971	79		
D7972	79		
D7980	79		
D7981	79		
D7982	79		
D7983	79		
D7990	80		
D7991	80		
D7995	80		
D7996	80		
D7997	80		
D7998	80		
D7999	80		

XI. Orthodontics

CDT Code	Page in CDT Manual Section		
D8010	81		
D8020	81		
D8030	81		
D8040	81		
D8050	82		
D8060	82		
D8070	82		
D8080	82		

CDT Code	Page in CDT Manual Section		Change Legend – ● = Addition ▲ = Revision
	1 - Current Version	2 - Change Summary	
D8090	82		
D8210	83		
D8220	83		
D8660	83		
D8670	83	.	
D8680	83		
D8690	83		
D8691	83		
D8692	83		
D8693	83	117	▲
D8694	83	117	●
D8999	83		

XII. Adjunctive General Services

CDT Code	1 - Current Version	2 - Change Summary	Change
D9110	85		
D9120	85		
D9210	85		
D9211	85		
D9212	85		
D9215	85		
D9220	85		
D9221	86		
D9230	86		
D9241	86		
D9242	86		
D9248	87		
D9310	87		
D9410	87		
D9420	87		
D9430	87		
D9440	87		
D9450	87		
D9610	88		
D9612	88		

| CDT Code | Page in CDT Manual Section | | Change Legend –
 ● = Addition
 ▲ = Revision |
	1 - Current Version	2 - Change Summary	
D9630	88		
D9910	88		
D9911	88		
D9920	88		
D9930	89		
D9940	89		
D9941	89		
D9942	89		
D9950	89		
D9951	89		
D9952	89		
D9970	89		
D9971	90		
D9972	90		
D9973	90		
D9974	90		
D9975	90		
D9985	90	119	●
D9999	90		

 © 2013 American Dental Association

5 Guide to the CDT Manual CD-ROM

ADA American Dental Association®

America's leading advocate for oral health

Guide to the CDT Manual CD-ROM

The CD-ROM included with this book contains the complete text of the American Dental Association's *CDT 2014: Current Dental Terminology* in electronic format.

Starting the CD-ROM

Insert the CD-ROM into your computer's CD-ROM drive. You will need to reinsert the CD-ROM each time you wish to run the program. The documents on this CD-ROM are provided in Adobe® PDF format. To view them, you will need **Adobe® Reader**. If you do not have this software, you can download it for free at *www.adobe.com/products/reader.html*. You can also install it on your computer (or test to see if you have it) from the CD-ROM menu.

- If you are using **Windows**, the menu may appear automatically after the title screen. If it does not, click on the Windows **Start** menu, select **Run**, and type in D:\cdt2014.exe (where "D" is you CD-ROM drive). The menu page will then appear. Just click on the heading of the document you'd like to view.

- If you are using a **Mac**, double-click on the "CDT 2014" CD icon on your desktop

Navigating Documents

Once opened, the PDF files will look like the pages of the CDT manual. You can turn on the **Bookmarks** feature of an open PDF document by clicking on the Bookmarks tab in the upper left corner. Each bookmark is a link to the corresponding section of the document. To get back to the Menu page, click on the **CDT icon** on the status bar at the bottom of the page, or close the Reader window. All PDF documents on the CD-ROM are searchable. There are two main ways to **locate a keyword or code** within the text of a document:

- To **Find** the next appearance of a term, hit Ctrl + F, type the search term and hit Enter. Or, choose Edit from the Menu bar, then Find. The Find function only looks for the term in the current document.

- To **Search** for all instances of a term in the document, hit Shift + Ctrl + F and type in the text. This Search function also allows you to search for the term in other documents on the CD-ROM or your computer. For help using Adobe® Reader, open the reader and select **Help** from the top menu bar at the top of your screen. You can also visit the Adobe® website at *www.adobe.com*.

Printing Documents

To print an open PDF document, click on the **Print** icon at the upper left of the page, or choose **File**, then **Print**. The entire chapter will print unless you specify Current Page or give a page range.

Exiting Program

To get out of the program, click on the **Close Window** icon (X at top right of the CD-ROM menu). You will see a message box with a question mark. Select "Exit program" and eject the CD-ROM from the drive.

Questions about CDT Content

For questions about dental procedure coding or claim submission, call the ADA Member Service Center at 800.621.8099. Support is available 8:30 a.m. to 5:00 p.m. CST, Monday through Friday.

Computer/CD Technical Support

For technical support regarding the *CDT 2014 CD-ROM*, call the ADA Technical Support Center toll free at 800.232.2165. Support is available 8:30 a.m. to 5:00 p.m. CST, Monday through Friday.